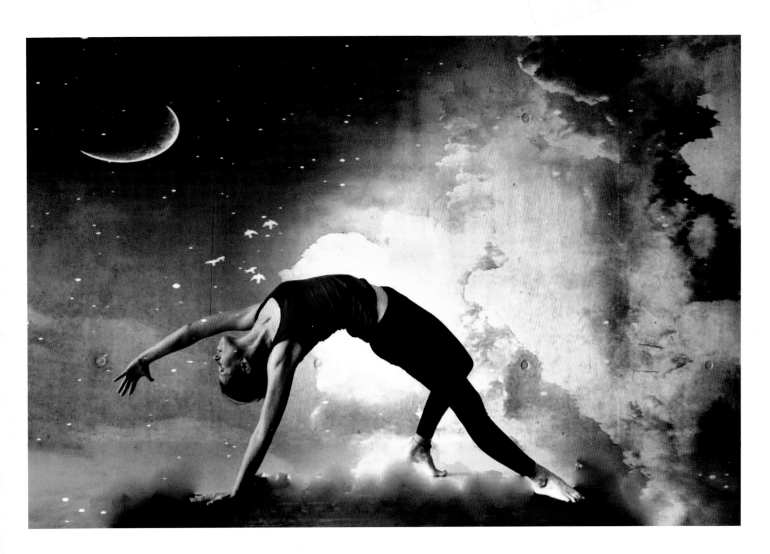

Yoga Fables

NATHALIE DOSWALD

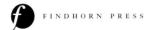
FINDHORN PRESS

Published in 2017 by Findhorn Press, Scotland

ISBN 978-1-84409-733-3

A CIP record for this title is available from the British Library.

Photos by Nathalie Doswald; except for pp. 12/13 (© Altaoosthuizen), p. 14 (© Lóránt Mátyás),
p. 56 (© Suppakij1017), p. 88 (© Lenka Šošolíková), cover background (© Madartists) –
all by Dreamstime.com
Model in photos: Chloé Bovay

Edited by Jacqui Lewis
Cover and interior design by
Geoff Green Book Design, CB24 4GL
Printed and bound in the EU

Disclaimer
The information in this book is given in good faith and is neither
intended to diagnose any physical or mental condition nor to serve
as a substitute for informed medical advice or care.
Please contact your health professional for medical advice and
treatment. Neither author nor publisher can be held liable by any
person for any loss or damage whatsoever which may arise from the
use of this book or any of the information therein.

Published by
Findhorn Press
117–121 High Street,
Forres IV36 1AB,
Scotland, UK

t +44 (0)1309 690582
f +44 (0)131 777 2711

e info@findhornpress.com
www.findhornpress.com

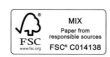

To my mentor, Louise Lloyd who inspired me to be myself; to Monika, Matea, Lucy, Debra and all my friends without whom this could have never happened; to Chloé Bovay for her beautiful asanas; to my family – birth family and soul family:

Thank you from the depths of my heart.

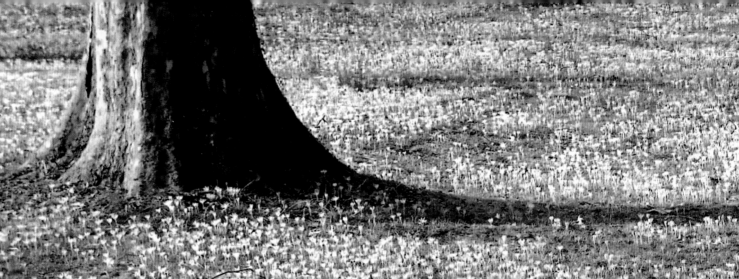

Contents

Introduction

O ur lives are stories told through our body and its movement. Our experiences and life choices are reflected in how we stand, how we move and in our health condition. Unexpressed emotion and trauma stays within the body until we allow it to be felt and released. Our bodies are a wealth of knowledge if only we would take the time to listen. Yet many of us use only our minds to understand ourselves and our stories, ignoring our bodies' wisdom.

Consciously embodying the story of our lives (rather than just thinking about it) allows us to understand ourselves at a deeper level. Fully embodying our experience of life gives us freedom to be ourselves. Yoga allows us to explore ourselves – body, mind, emotions and spirit – and learn to live fully embodied.

Personal growth and development can sometimes feel painful and serious: life experiences can be traumatic and feelings, so often repressed, can be difficult to deal with. Yet learning and life do not have to always be so. Playfulness, fun and creativity also allow us to learn and develop. Learning to love our bodies and have fun with them, as they are in this moment, gives us space to be; and from that place of being we grow.

Yoga Fables aims to awaken creativity and fun in the practice of yoga and in the practice of self-discovery through embodying stories so as to access our stories and our own innate wisdom.

This book arose from my own personal yoga practice, which helped me recover from 20 years of depression and anorexia due to trauma. Trauma can sap creativity and problem-solving, as well as connection to the body and oneself. Coming to a place of playfulness and connecting with my inner child allowed me to come back home to myself, learn to love my body and tap into my inner wisdom.

While we may not all have mental health problems, many of us are dissatisfied with ourselves, our bodies and our lives, or have lived through difficult times. This dissatisfaction and hardship often translate into us mistreating ourselves in some way, e.g. self-criticism, overwork or addictions, in an effort to cope and survive. Coming back to a place of self-nurture and fun can restore our balance and bring us back in touch with who we really are.

A Note on Sequences

Each of the sequences here follows a fable. It does so organically and globally while still taking into account the principles of good yoga sequencing. Each sequence contains a warm-up, an active phase and a cool-down phase so as to gradually open the body and then bring it back to stillness and relaxation. To allow for this important process, not every single posture in a sequence will have meaning for the story. The story and the sequence may be taken as a whole, interacting together to provide opportunities for insight.

Within each sequence, ensure that your transitions between poses are fluid and careful. There are suggestions for modifications of the poses, but feel free to modify according to your need and capability. At the back of the book, you will find some safety guidelines (e.g. advice for pregnancy, back problems, etc.) but this is no substitute for listening to your body (and a qualified health practitioner).

And most importantly, have fun. There is fun to be had in yoga just as in life. These stories and sequences are here for each and every reader to interpret and explore as they wish.

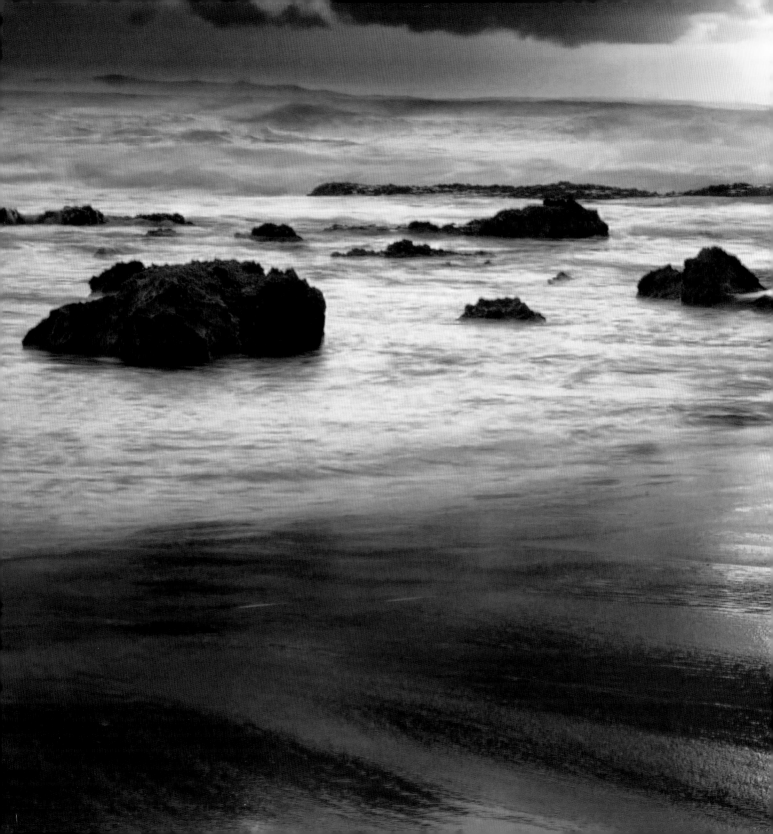

Sun Salutations and Common Postures

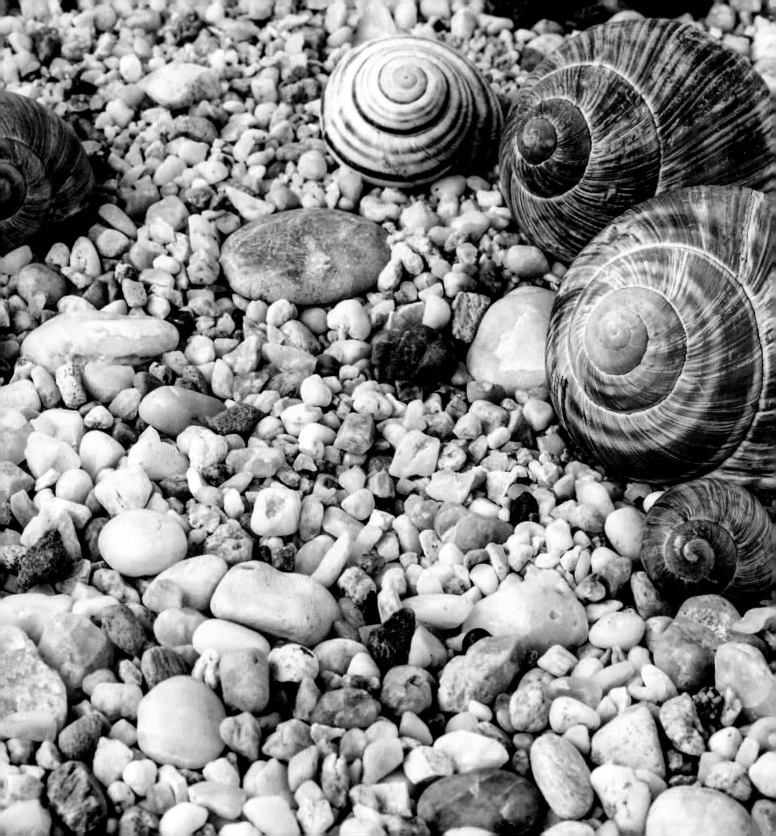

Sun Salutations

Sun salutations feature often in the practices throughout this book.
Familiarise yourself with them beforehand, if you like.

Classical sun salutation

Poses 1–12 represent one half of the sun salutation, stepping back with the right foot in position 4 and stepping forward with the right foot in position 9. The second half is done with the left foot leading.

Indicated are which breath (inhale or exhale) to take with the movement. It is OK to add more breaths in each pose. It can also be nice to hold position 8 (Downward dog) for a few breaths to check in with your body and breath.

1. Exhale

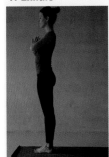

Hands in prayer

2. Inhale

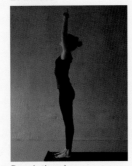

Reach the sky

3. Exhale

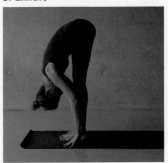

Standing forward fold

Yoga Fables

4. Inhale

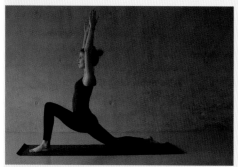

Crescent moon lunge

5. Hold for 1 full breath

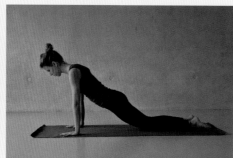

Half plank

6. Exhale

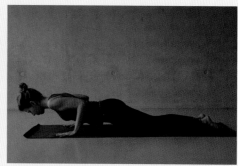

Half four-limbed staff

7. Inhale

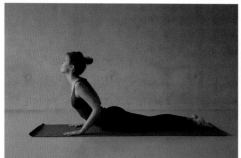

Cobra

8. Exhale

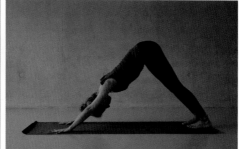

Downward dog

9. Inhale

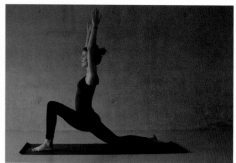

Crescent moon lunge

10. Exhale

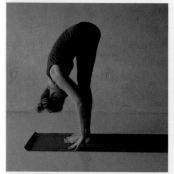

Standing forward fold

11. Inhale

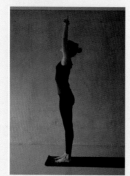

Reach the sky

12. Exhale

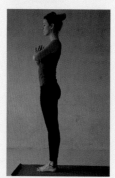

Hands in prayer

Variation A (or Sun A)

1. Exhale

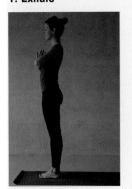

Hands in prayer

2. Inhale

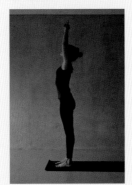

Reach the sky

3. Exhale

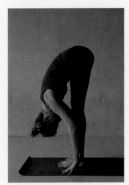

Standing forward fold

4. Inhale

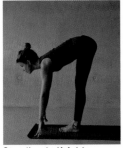

Standing half-fold

5. Hold for 1 full breath

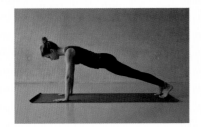

Plank

6. Exhale

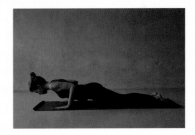

Half four-limbed staff

7. Inhale

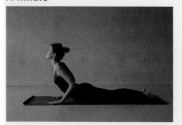

Cobra

8. Exhale

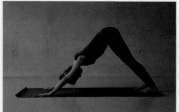

Downward dog

9. Inhale

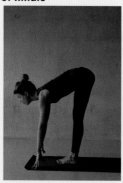

Standing half-fold

10. Exhale

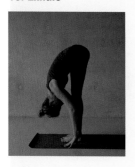

Standing forward fold

11. Inhale

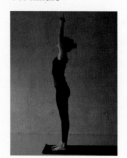

Reach the sky

12. Exhale

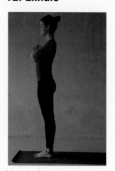

Hands in prayer

Variation B (or Sun B)

1. Exhale

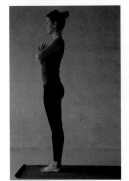

Hands in prayer

2. Inhale

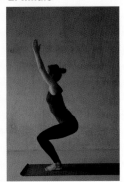

Fierce pose

3. Exhale

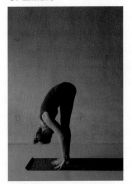

Standing forward fold

4. Inhale

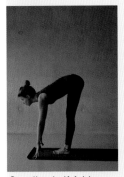

Standing half-fold

5. Hold for 1 full breath

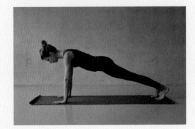

Plank

6. Exhale

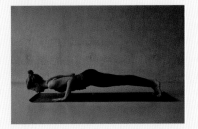

Four-limbed staff

7. Inhale

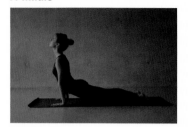

Upward dog

8. Exhale

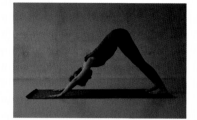

Downward dog

9. Inhale

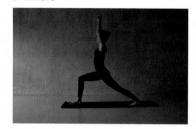

Warrior I (right leg front)

10. Repeat 5–8

11. Inhale

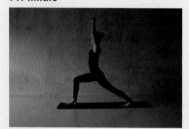

Warrior I (left leg front)

12. Repeat 5–8

13. Inhale

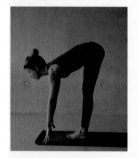

Standing half-fold

14. Exhale

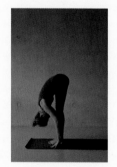

Standing forward fold

15. Inhale

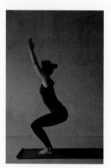

Fierce pose

16. Exhale

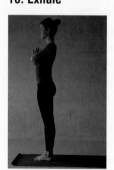

Hands in prayer

Vinyasa

1.Inhale

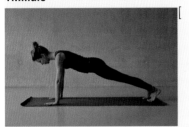

Plank

2. Exhale

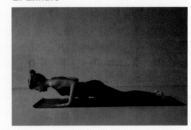

Half four-limbed staff

3. Inhale

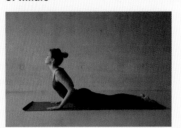

Cobra

Common Postures

Alternate arms and legs

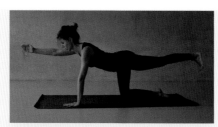

Extend one leg and opposite arm, keeping your core tight.

Bharadvaja's twist

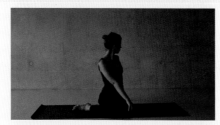

Sitting with both feet pointing to one side, ensure that hips are level. Sit one buttock on cushion if necessary to level hips. Keep spine tall as you twist away from your feet.

Bridge

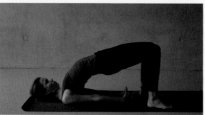

With feet parallel, lift hips up keeping knees in line with your hips. You can clasp your hands behind back.

Cat–cow

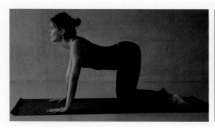 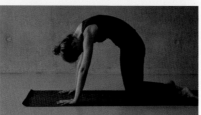

Inhale on A and exhale on B.

Child pose

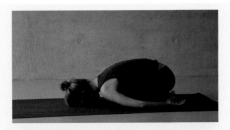

If your head does not reach the floor, you can place it on your stacked hands or fists.

Child pose extended

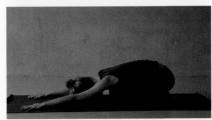

Stretch the arms while keeping the shoulders soft.

Cobra

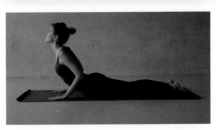

Keep lower back long by pressing pubic bone to floor and keeping the core tight. Keep all toe nails pressing into the ground and open upper chest with elbows close to ribcage.

Crescent moon lunge

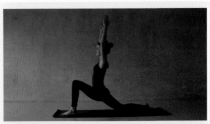

Ensure that the front knee does not collapse inwards towards the body's midline.

Downward dog

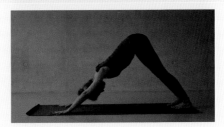

Press hips up and back. Feet hip-width apart or more. Knees can be bent to help lengthen your spine. It's fine if heels do not touch the floor.

Downward dog open leg

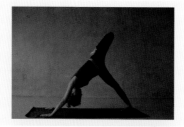

From downward dog, lift one leg up, open at the hip, bending the knee.

Downward dog split

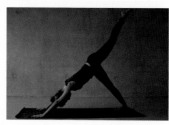

From downward dog, lift one leg up.

Dynamic cat

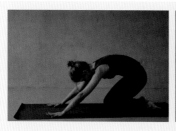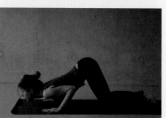

Starting on all fours, A exhale, rounding back and sitting on heels, B inhale, sweeping forward chin towards floor, coming back to all fours. Repeat.

Eye of needle

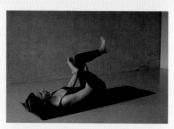

The feet should be flexed.

Fish

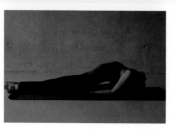

Hands under buttocks with palms on the mat. Elbows tight against ribcage. Lift on to elbows and arch back and neck, gently resting head on the mat.

Five-pointed star

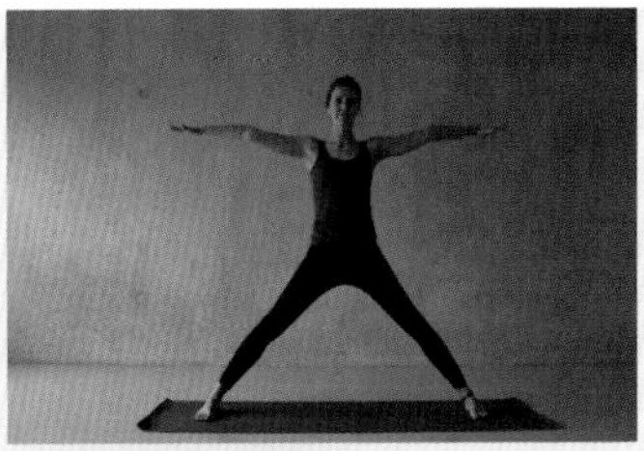

Extend through arms, legs and crown of the head.

Fierce pose

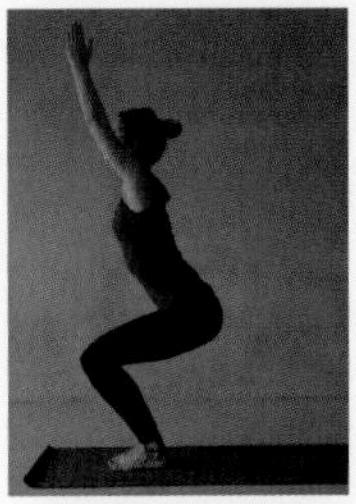

Feet and knees together, sit back, keeping spine long.

Gate pose

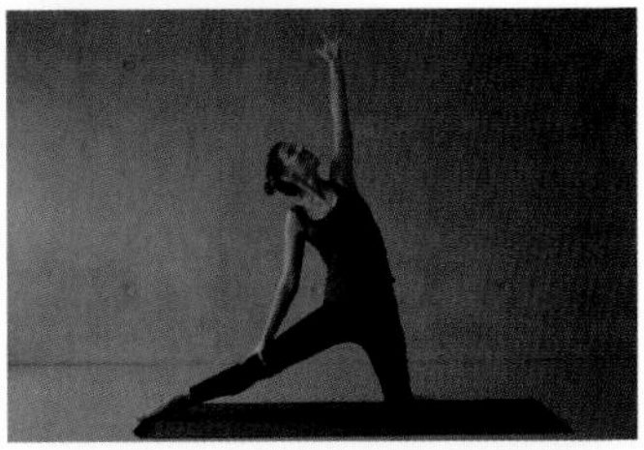

Keep hips facing front. Flex sideways over extended leg. Can have the foot of the extended leg flexed (toes up) instead of toes towards the floor.

Half lord of the fishes

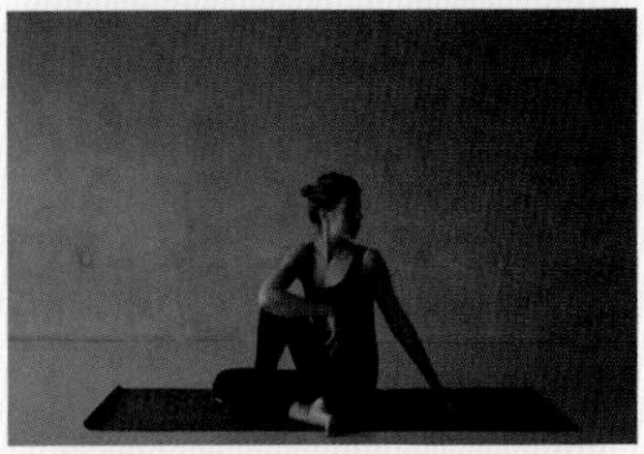

Can leave bottom leg straight instead of folded back. Root into sit bones, and keep spine long as you twist towards your bent knee.

Happy baby pose

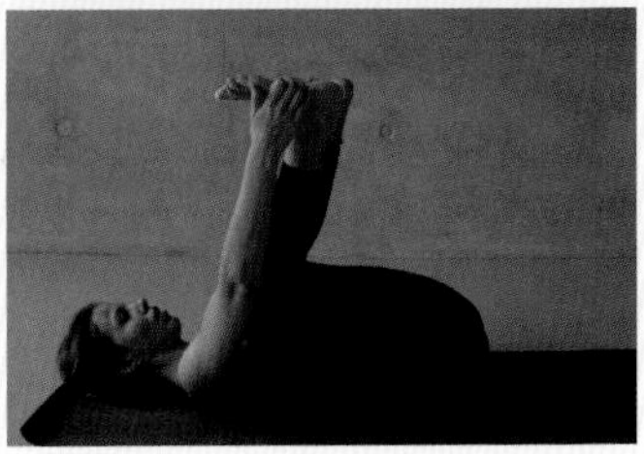

Grasp feet or shins and keep pelvis on floor.

Lizard

No need to lower elbows to the floor if very uncomfortable. Can also lift back knee off floor.

Locust

Extend in length rather than height. Keep hips planted and core tight. Can also extend arms forward. Inhale lifting, exhale down.

Low lunge twist up

Ensure that the front knee does not collapse inwards towards the body's midline. Keep chest open as you twist.

Low lunge prayer twist

Ensure that the front knee does not collapse inwards towards the body's midline. Keep chest open as you twist.

Low lunge quad stretch

Ensure that the front knee does not collapse inwards towards the body's midline.

Lunge runner's

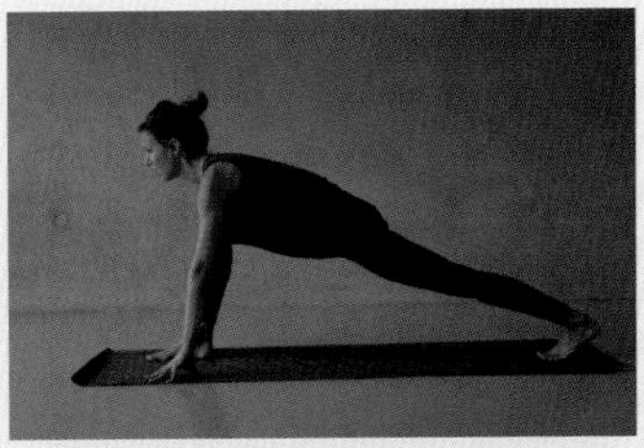

Press into heel to lengthen.

Lunge with twist up

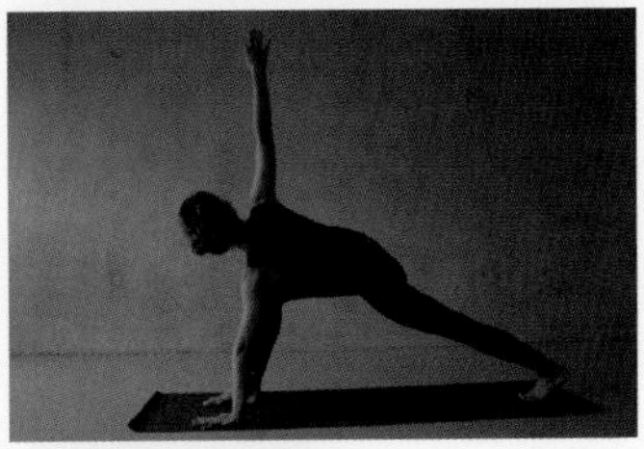

Keep chest open as you twist towards your knee.

Mountain pose

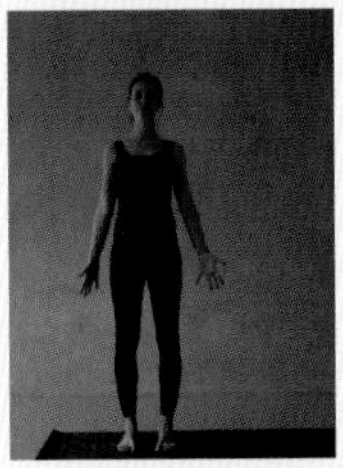

Standing tall, press down into four corners of feet. Squeeze thighs towards each other. Hands by your sides extending through fingers.

Plank

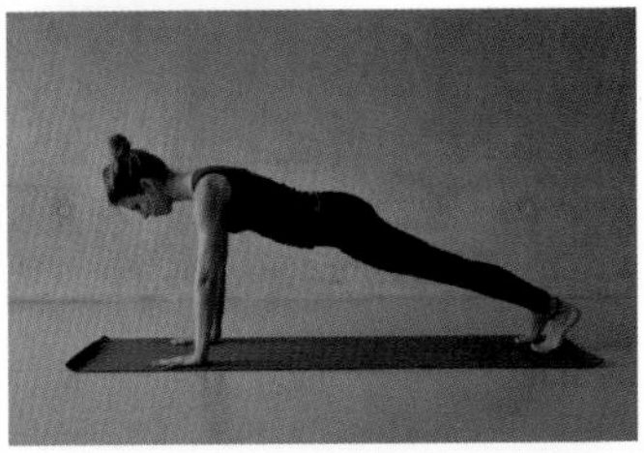

Core tight. For half plank, have knees on floor.

Plough

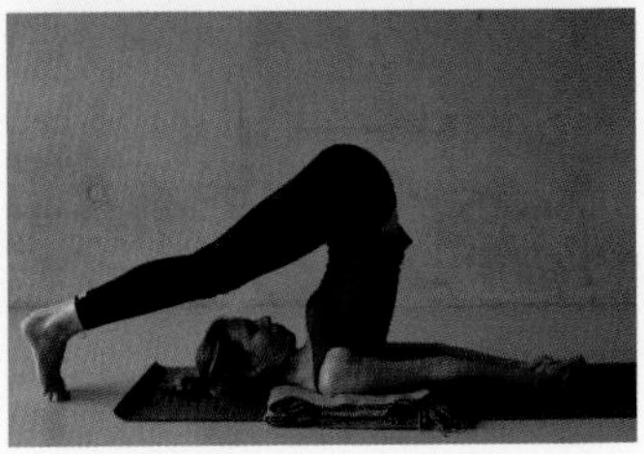

Can have shoulders supported by a blanket as shown to stress the neck less.

**Pyramid
(with reverse prayer)**

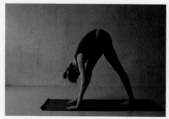 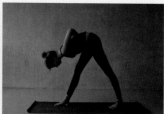

Ensure that hips are level. Can leave front knee slightly bent. For arms in reverse prayer, palms together behind back or just crossed behind, holding elbows.

Relaxation

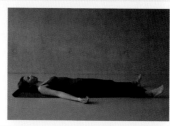

Can have knees bent instead.

Revolved fierce pose

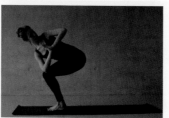

Ensure both knees are same level. Twist to one side. Can extend arms instead of having them in prayer

Revolved gate

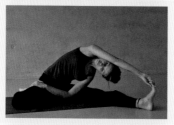

Keep both sit bones grounded and side ribs facing the sky. If bent knee uncomfortable with foot pointing backwards, do revolved head to knee pose instead.

Revolved head to knee

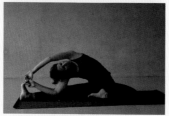

Keep both sit bones grounded and side ribs facing sky. Can bend the extended leg if necessary.

Seated forward fold

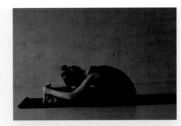

Keep both sit bones grounded. Fold from the hips. Can bend the knees if lower back is uncomfortable.

Seated head to knee forward bend

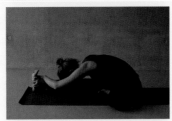

Keep both sit bones grounded. Fold from the hips over extended leg. Can bend the knee if lower back is uncomfortable.

Seated side stretch

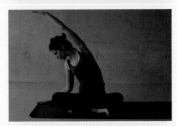

Keep both sit bones grounded and side ribs facing the sky as you bend.

Seated twist

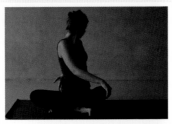

Keep both sit bones grounded, spine tall and chest open as you twist.

Shoulder stand

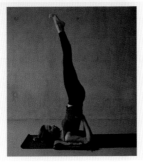

Have arms and shoulders on a blanket to protect the neck. Can also do half shoulder stand, where legs are angled slightly over head to make body into a C-shape.

Side angle

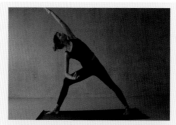

Ensure that knee does not go past the ankle and that knee is tracking second toe. Keep weight even on both feet. Can also place hand on floor inside the leg, if possible, instead of having elbow on the thigh.

Side plank

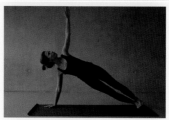

Hand below shoulder, fingers spread. Keep hips high. Can also place top foot on floor in front to stabilise the posture.

Sphinx

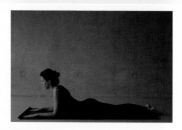

Hips on floor, arms at right angle, core tight, open chest.

Staff pose

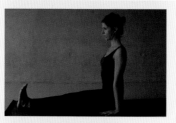

Keep both sit bones grounded and spine tall.

Standing hand to foot pose – straight

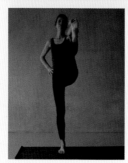

To keep back straight, can just hold bent knee towards chest instead.

Standing hand to foot pose – open to the side

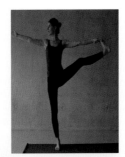

To keep back straight, can just hold bent knee towards chest and then open to the side instead.

Standing forward fold (with arms behind)

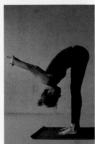 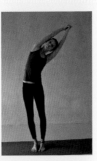

Fold from the hips. Bend knees if necessary. In the arms-clasped version, the arms may not lift much from back.

Standing side bend

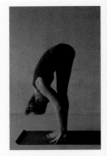

Keep both feet anchored with equal weight as you bend.

Standing twist

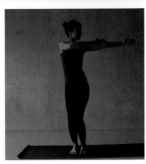

Keep both feet anchored with equal weight as you twist.

Supine butterfly

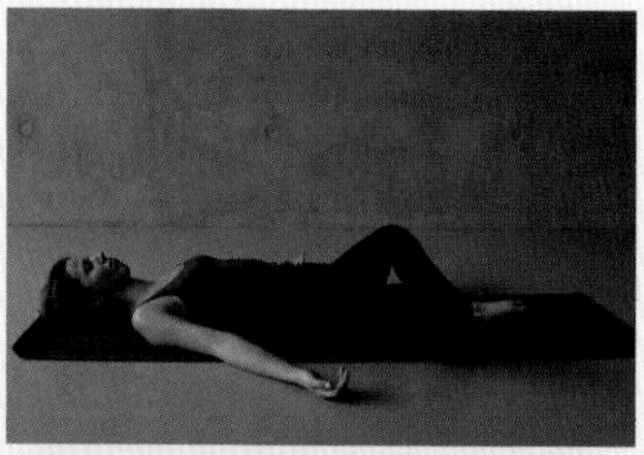

Feet together with knees opening to the side.

Supine head to one knee

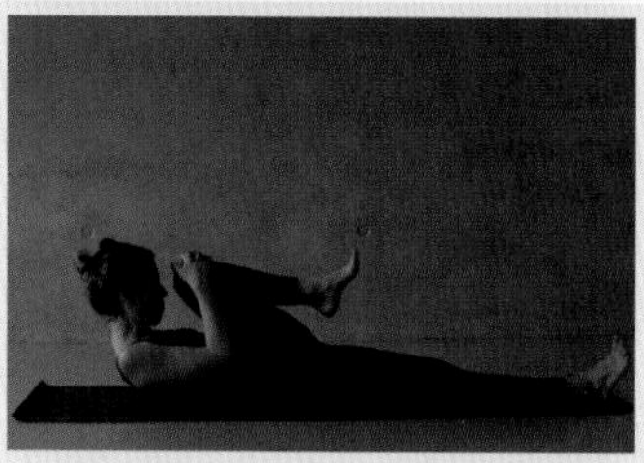

Keep extended leg pressing down and core tight as you bring forehead to knee.

Supine knees to chest

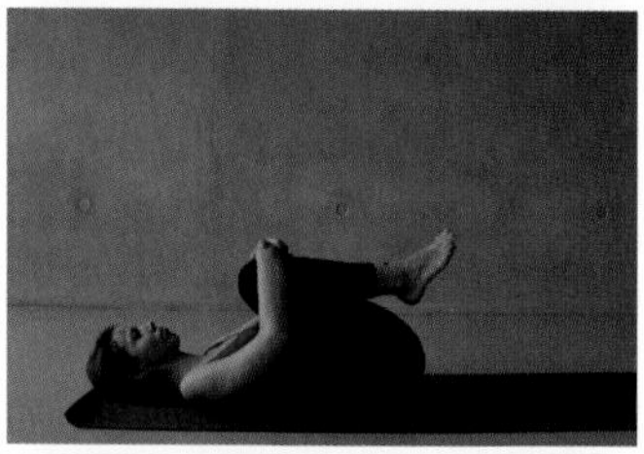

Press hips into the floor to lengthen the spine.

Supine twist

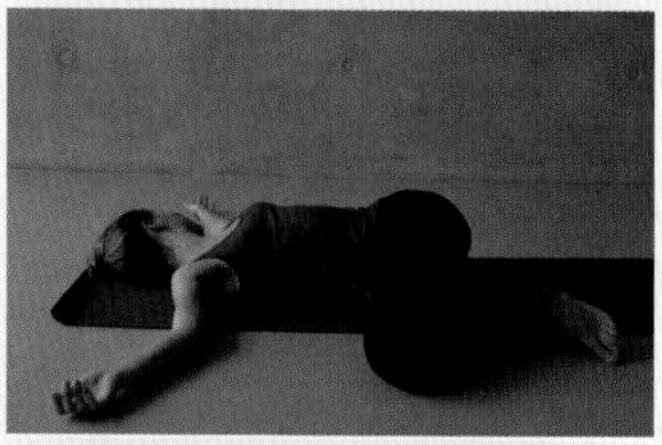

Keep both shoulders on the floor.

Tree

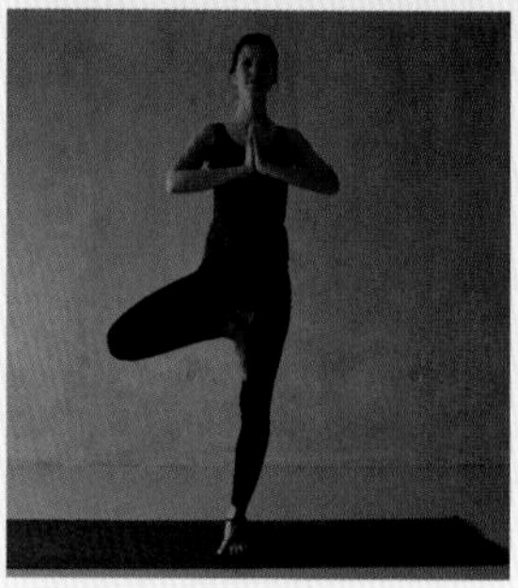

Can either rest lifted foot on floor near ankle, on shin or on thigh (not on knee).
Can also lift hands overhead.

Tree side

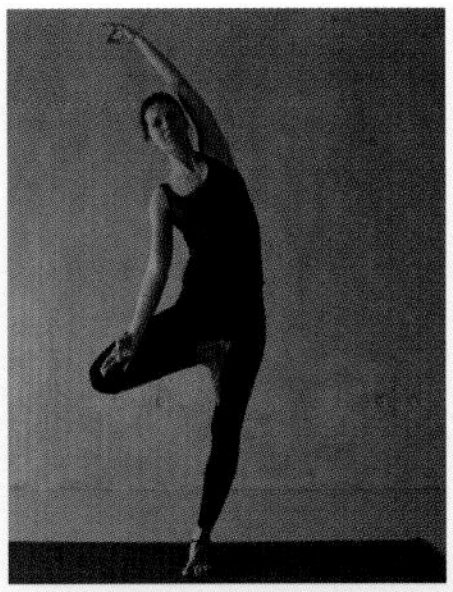

Lifted foot can rest either on floor near ankle, on shin or on thigh (not on knee).

Triangle

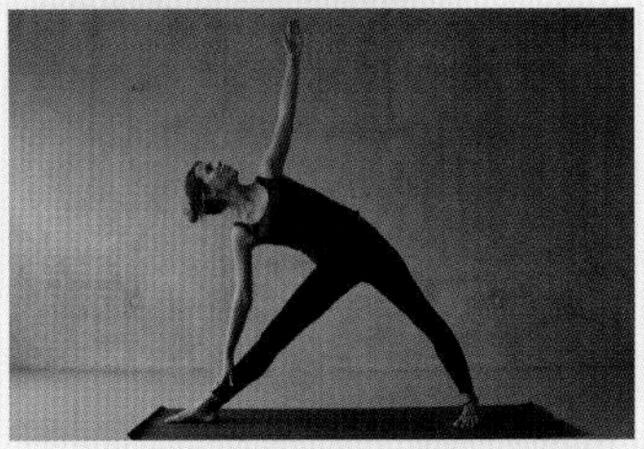

Push both hips back as you fold and open the chest with side ribs facing sky. Don't go down too far if you find chest facing floor. Can have top arm on hip rather than extended.

Warrior I

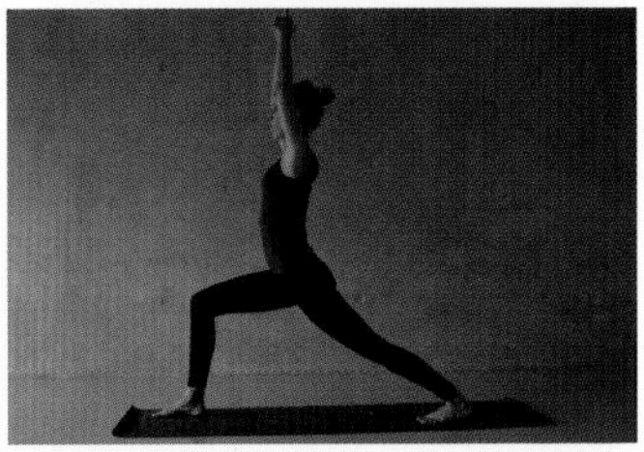

Ensure that knee does not collapse inwards towards the body's midline and does not go over ankle. Your hips and torso are facing the front of your mat.

Warrior II

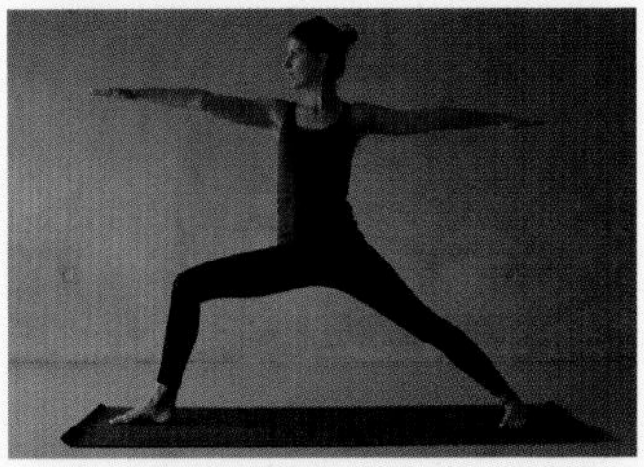

Ensure that knee does not go over ankle and that knee is tracking second toe. Torso is open to the side.

Warrior III

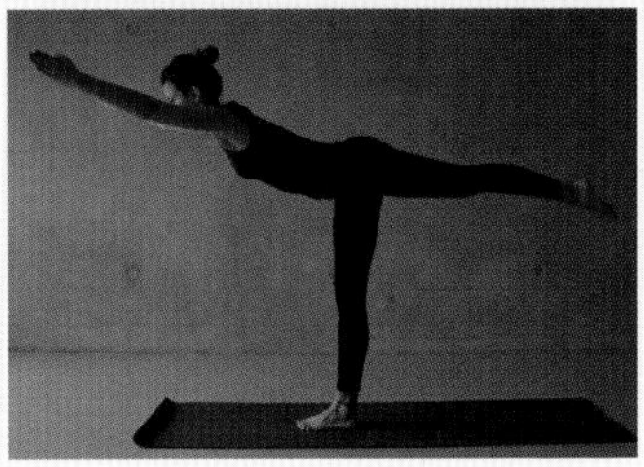

Keep both hips level and core tight. Having hands on hips rather than ahead makes this pose easier.

Humble warrior

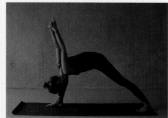

From warrior I, fold from the hips. Hands clasped behind. Arms may not lift much off your back.

Warrior reverse

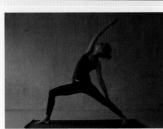

From warrior II, arch back.

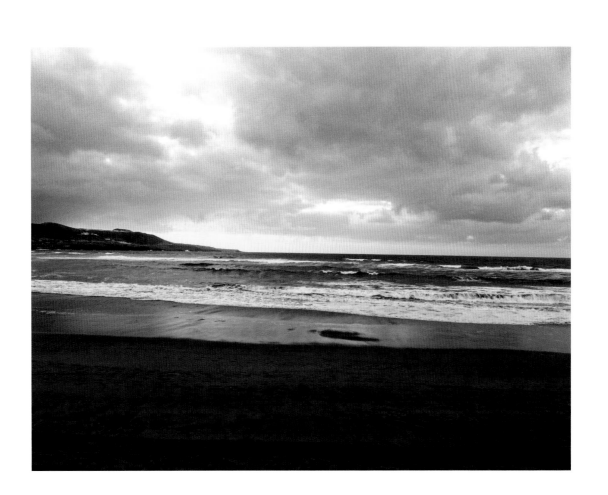

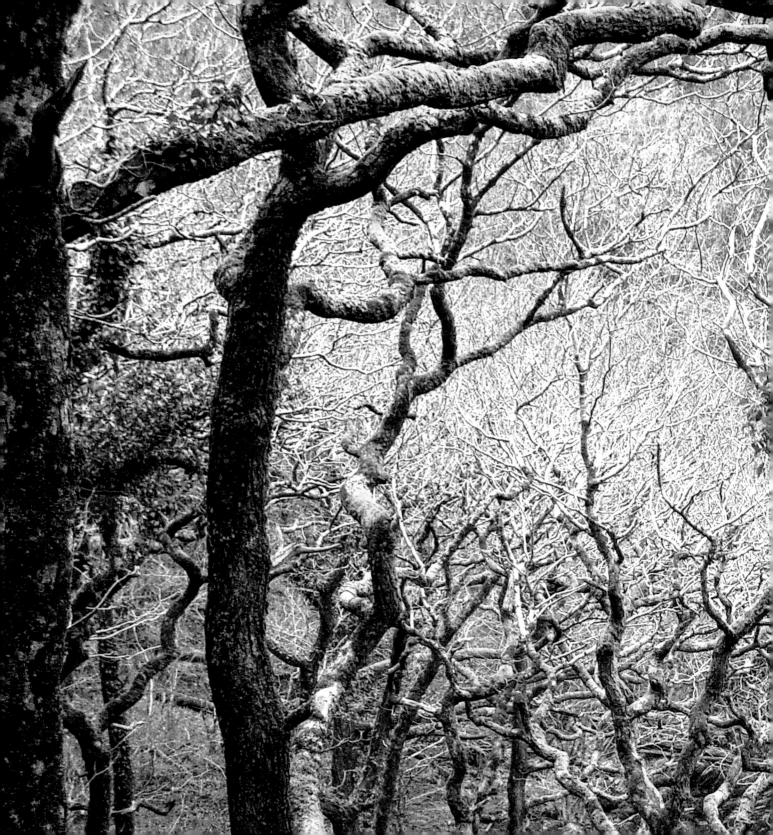

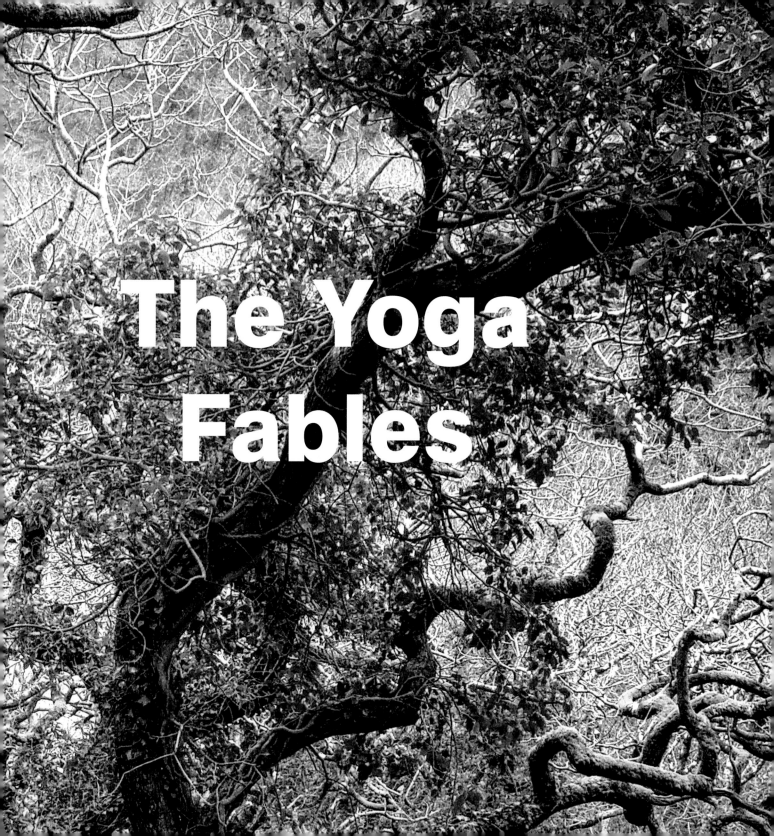

The Yoga Fables

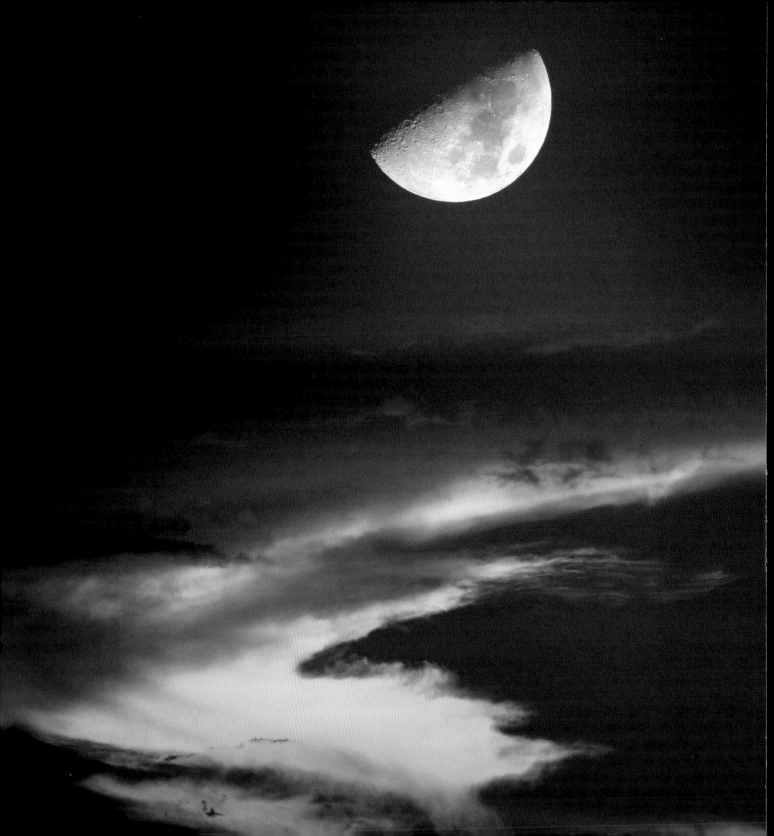

The Warrior Seeking the Moon

'Let the waters settle and you will see the moon and stars mirrored in your being.'

Rumi

'Living life without hope is like forgetting the moonshine simply
because it is hidden behind a passing cloud.'

Unknown

Up on a high windy outcrop, a warrior sat under a tree waiting for the full moon to appear. He waited patiently for 30 nights and days. His patience started to wear thin as endless clouds obscured the night. And so he prayed, unheard, to the forever clouded sky.

Frustration set in. The mountain stood stoic as he begged and implored under the tree. His emotions flowed and reached a peak of rage. At times he found himself near madness, willing the clouds to move so he could see the moon. Tired and despairing, he sank down to his knees, his arms outstretched on the rocky ground.

Within his cold despair and frustration, he felt underneath his hand something smooth, nearly warm — a root from the tree. Looking up at the tree, he smiled. Despite his stormy emotions, despite the swirling winds around, the tree stood solid, stately and wise.

Courage swelled in his breast as he realised he knew what he should do. The tree remained unwavering, and so the warrior decided he should be. And so he stood, centred and grounded as a tree.

The clouds shifted slowly, revealing light from the moon. The warrior stirred, excited. Soon he would see the full moon, his patience rewarded. The wind swept the sky clear, leaving hanging a large yellow half-moon in a star-studded sky. Disappointment flooded the warrior. As floodwaters rose in his heart, his rage stormed again.

His rage eventually abated, turning into grief at what seemed lost. Then, looking up to the stars, he asked for hope, courage and faith while offering his heart to the sky.

Looking back at the half-moon, his grief dissolved as he melted into its beauty. Drinking in the detail and nuances of the moon, he saw a faint outline making the moon whole. Light flickered in his mind as he realised that even though half the moon was in shadow, the full moon was in fact there. Light filled his mind as he realised that even though it had been covered by clouds, the full moon was always there.

The warrior left the windy outcrop and went home. He never sought the moon again because he knew in his heart that it was always there.

Sequence: The Warrior Seeking the Moon

The warrior is patiently waiting for the full moon to appear.

1. Seated

2. Seated neck stretch

3. Seated side bend

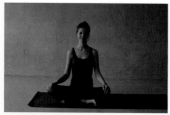

Comfortable seated position. Sit bones are rooted in the earth and spine is long. Feel your breath.

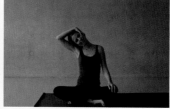

In the seated position, tilt head to one side using your hand gently on the head.
Both sides

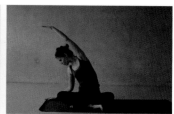

Keep both sit bones grounded and side ribs facing the sky as you bend.
Both sides

4. Seated twist

His patience starts to fray…

5. Cat-cow

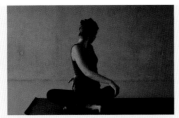

Keep both sit bones grounded and chest open as you twist.
Both sides

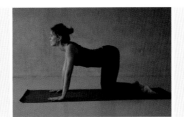

Inhale

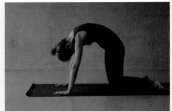

Exhale
3–6 times

6. Thread the needle

The warrior prays…

7. Quarter dog

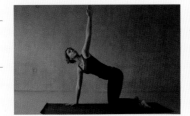

Inhale

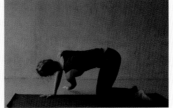

Exhale
3–6 times on both sides

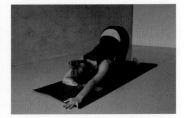

Both sides

to the sky.

8. Crescent moon lunge

9. Downward dog

10. Repeat 8–9, other side.

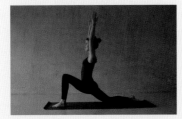

Ensure that the front knee does not collapse inwards towards the body's midline.

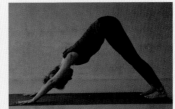

Press hips up and back. Feet hip-width apart or more. Knees can be bent to help lengthen your spine. It's fine if heels do not touch the floor.

Repeat 8–9, other side

11. Standing forward fold

The mountain stood stoic as...

12. Mountain prayer

...the warrior begged

13. Reach the sky

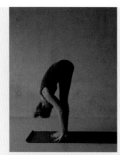

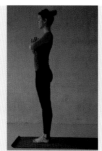

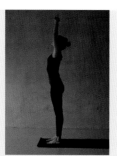

Step feet to front of mat. Fold from the hips. Bend knees if necessary.

Standing tall, press down into four corners of feet. Squeeze thighs towards each other. Hands in prayer in front of heart.

The following sequence 14–31: Do whole sequence on one side with right leg standing first (lifting left leg); and right arm holding the side plank. Then do the other side as indicated below.

...and implored...

14. Mountain prayer

under the tree.

15. Tree

16. Tree side with earth mudra

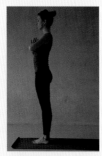

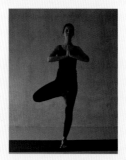

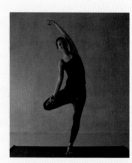

Standing tall, press down into four corners of feet. Squeeze thighs towards each other. Hands in prayer in front of heart.

Can either rest lifted foot on floor near ankle, on shin or on thigh (not on knee). Can also lift hands overhead.

From Tree, place one hand on thigh and lift the other. For earth mudra: bring your thumb to your ring (fourth) finger.

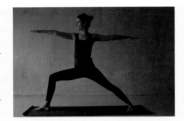 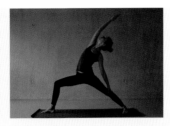 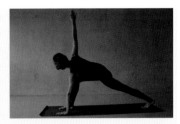

Ensure that knee is tracking second toe. Torso is open to side.

From warrior II, arch back on an inhale.

Keep chest open as you twist towards your knee.

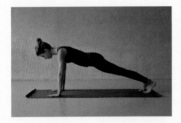 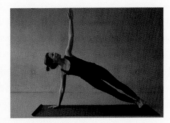 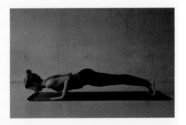

Core tight. (For crunches, bring one knee towards chest, then change sides.)

Hand below shoulder, fingers spread. Keep hips high. Can also place top foot on floor in front to stabilise the posture.

From plank lower toward floor either body as one (as shown); alternative; lower first knees and then chest.

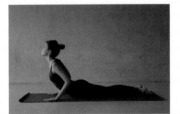 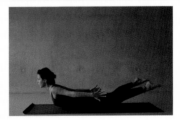 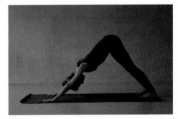

Keep lower back long by pressing pubic bone to floor and keep the core tight. Keep all toenails pressing into the ground and open upper chest with elbows close to ribcage.

Inhale to lift and exhale down.

(Can add knee crunches by bringing right knee to right elbow, left elbow and in between hands. Switch sides.)

26. Downward dog open leg

At times he found himself near madness, willing the clouds to move so he could see the moon.

27. Wildthing

28. Side plank

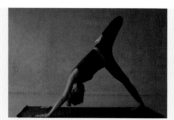

From downward dog, lift one leg up, open at the hip, bending the knee.

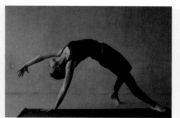

From downward dog open leg, allow lifted leg to drop behind to the floor. Press hips up and arch back.

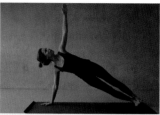

Hand below shoulder, fingers spread. Keep hips high. Can also place top foot on floor in front to stabilise the posture.

29. Downward dog (or vinyasa to downward dog)

30. Standing forward fold

31. Standing hands in prayer

32. Repeat 14–29 on other side. From 29 move to 33.

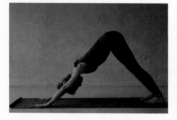

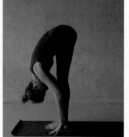

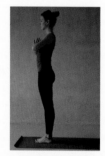

Repeat 14–29 on other side. From 29 move to 33.

The warrior sinks to the ground, cold with despair, feels the ground and the roots of the tree under his hands.

33. Child pose extended

Courage spreads through the warrior.

34. Thunderbolt pose with Ganesh mudra

The warrior knows his way.

35. Gate pose

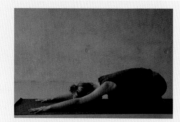

Sit on heels with arms outstretched.

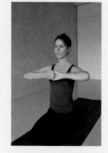

Sit on heels if OK with knees; otherwise sit however is comfortable. Left palm closest to chest. Exhale pull arms apart, keeping hands together, inhale release six times. Then put both hands on heart.

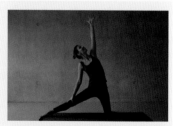

Keep hips facing front. Flex sideways over extended leg. Can have the foot of the extended leg flexed (toes up) instead of toes towards the floor. Both sides.Then roll up to standing.

The following sequence 36 to 41. Do whole sequence on one side with right leg standing (lifting left leg); and right arm holding the side plank. Then do the other side as indicated below.

36. Mountain pose

The warrior stands solid...

37. Standing hand to foot pose – straight and open to the side

...like a tree.

38. Tree

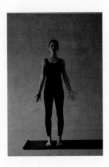 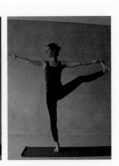 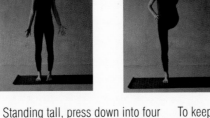 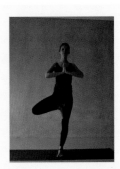

Standing tall, press down into four corners of feet. Squeeze thighs towards each other. Hands by your sides extending through fingers.

To keep back straight, can just hold bent knee towards chest and then open to the side instead.

Can either rest lifted foot on floor near ankle, on shin or on thigh (not on knee). Can also lift hands overhead.

The warrior stirred, excited, as the clouds moved...

39. Warrior II

...to reveal a magnificent half-moon.

40. Half moon

Disappointment and rage flooded the warrior.

41. Repeat 17–31

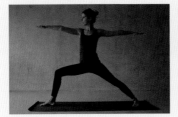 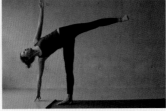

From Tree, step back lifted leg into warrior II.

From warrior II, take weight onto front leg and reach down towards floor with front hand. Back leg lifts. Push through both feet, opening torso to the side.

Repeat sequence 17–31.

42. Repeat 36–41 on the other side. Then roll down to kneeling.

His rage eventually abated, turning into grief at what seemed lost.

43. Child pose

The warrior asks for hope, courage and faith…

44. Thunderbolt pose with Ganesh mudra

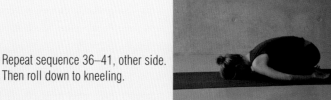
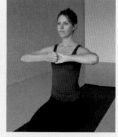

Repeat sequence 36–41, other side. Then roll down to kneeling.

Right palm closest to chest. Exhale pull arms apart keeping hands together, inhale release six times. Then put both hands on heart.

…offering his heart to the sky.

45. Camel

The warrior gazes at the moon, really seeing it for the first time.

46. Cobbler's pose

Light flickers as he realises…

47. Seated head to knee forward bend

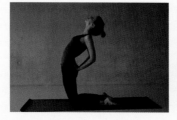
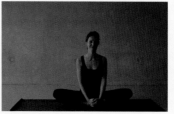
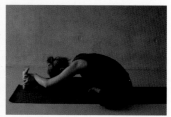

Keep hips pressing forward, chest open, lower back long. Should feel no pinching in lower back. To advance pose, can bring hands to heels rather than back.
Fold into child pose before moving to next pose.

Sit with soles of the feet together close to hips and keep back straight.

Keep both sit bones grounded. Fold from the hips over extended leg. Can bend the knee if lower back is uncomfortable.

…the full moon is always there.

48. Half lord of the fishes

49. Repeat 47–48, other side

The warrior goes home…

50. Supine knees to chest

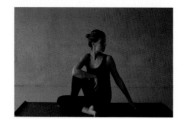
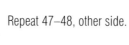
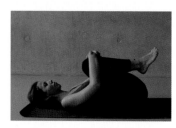

Can leave bottom leg straight instead of folded back. Root into sit bones, and keep spine long as you twist towards your bent knee.

Repeat 47–48, other side.

Press hips into the floor to lengthen the spine.

...happy because...

51. Happy baby pose

...he knows and trusts the moon is always there.

52. Relaxation

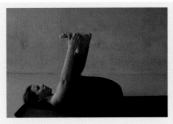 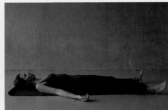

Grasp feet or shins and keep pelvis on floor.   Can have knees bent.

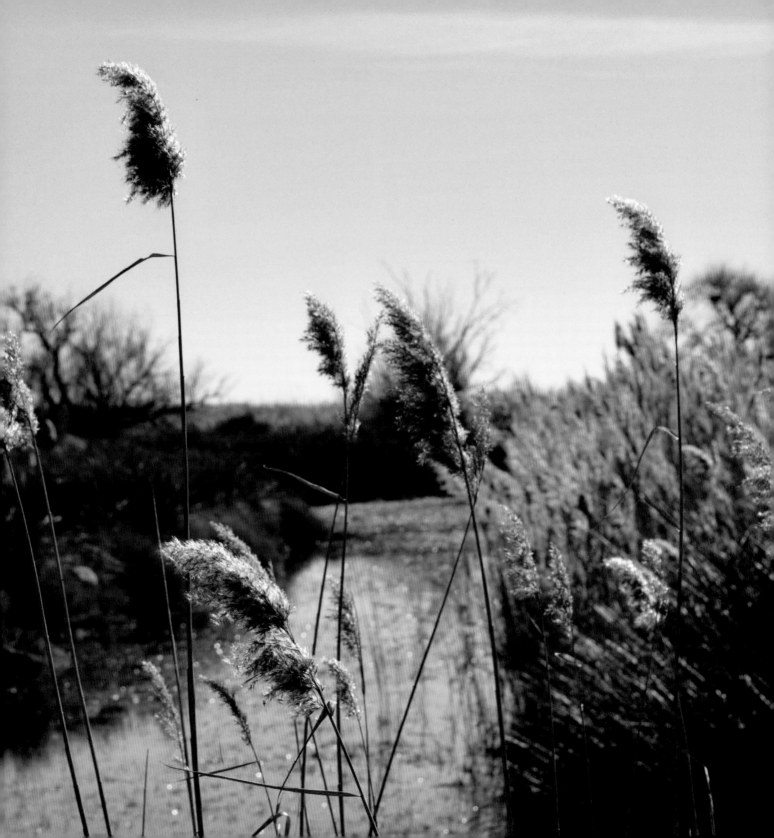

The Cobra and the Frog

'It's the ego that wants to feel important; the consciousness doesn't care.
The consciousness simply is.'

Gabriel Picazo

'When you are content to be simply yourself and don't compare or compete,
everyone will respect you.'

Lao Tzu

Deep in the old forest, animals stirred and scurried away. They were fearful not of the king of the forest, the old lion, but of the mighty cobra. The royal cobra was a fearsome beast full of self-importance. He dominated all: from the wild dogs to the lowly lizard. His bite was deadly and only complete abjection could save those that crossed his path.

One day, however, the cobra's path was not clear. There in the middle of the path stood an ordinary frog. The cobra reared higher, imposingly. The frog did not cower or retreat.

'Why do you not run away? Why do you not cower? Do you not fear me?' asked the cobra, taken aback.

'Why should I?' asked the frog.

'Because I am fearsome,' the cobra replied. 'My venom can injure any warrior who strides in this forest. The strength of my supple body can break the neck of a swan.'

'Well,' replied the frog casually, 'I have hopped away from arrows from the boys' bows.'

The cobra snorted. 'My mouth can engulf an entire child!'

'Maybe you are mighty; but only until you meet those that are mightier than you,' retorted the frog as a pigeon swooped down on the cobra's head, momentarily blinding him. The king lion roared and swiped the cobra from the side. He flew into the air, twisting and tumbling before landing outstretched on the ground.

Hopping back to his pond, the frog called back to the stricken cobra, *'I at least know that I am just a frog.'*

His pride wounded more than anything else, the cobra reflected on himself, mulling over the frog's words. Maybe he was no more or less than anyone else.

Sequence: The Cobra and the Frog

Deep in the old forest…

1. Thunderbolt pose

…animals stirred…

2. Side stretch

3. Twist

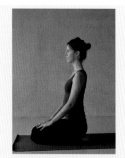 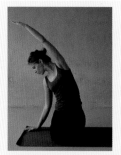 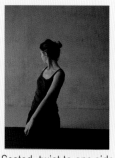

Sit on heels. If not comfortable sit cross-legged.

Seated, lift one arm up and stretch to the side.
Both sides.

Seated, twist to one side.

Both sides.

…and scurried away.

4. Cat–cow

They were fearful not of the old lion…

5. Lion

6. Half plank

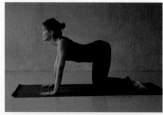 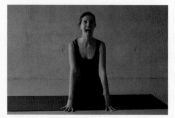 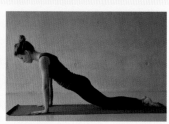

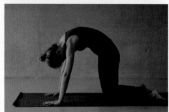

↑ Sit on heels, stick tongue out and roar!

← Inhale on A and exhale on B.

3–6 times

Core tight

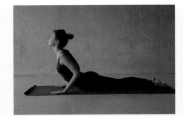 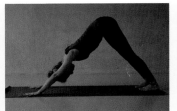 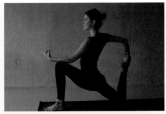

Keep lower back long by pressing pubic bone to floor and keep core tight. Keep all toenails pressing into the ground and open upper chest with elbows close to ribcage.

Press hips up and back. Feet hip-width apart or more. Knees can be bent to help lengthen your spine. It's fine if heels do not touch the floor.

Ensure that the front knee does not collapse inwards towards the body's midline. If cannot grasp back foot or knee is uncomfortable, keep back foot on the floor.

Repeat sequence 8–9, other side.

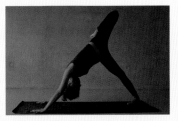 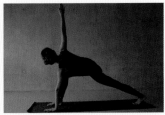

From downward dog, lift one leg up, open at the hip, bending the knee. Place lifted leg forward into next pose.

Keep chest open as you twist towards your knee.

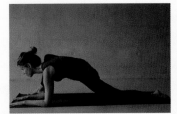 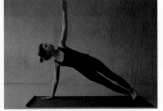 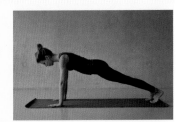

No need to lower elbows to the floor if very uncomfortable. Can also lift back knee off floor.

Hand below shoulder, fingers spread. Keep hips high. Can also place top foot on floor in front to stabilise the posture.

Core tight.

16. Cobra

Only complete abjection…

17. Child pose extended

18. Downward dog

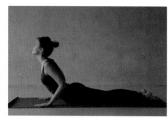
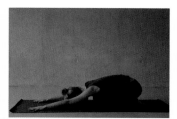
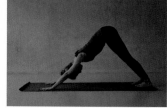

Keep lower back long by pressing pubic bone to floor and core tight. Keep all toenails pressing into the ground and open upper chest with elbows close to ribcage.

Press hips up and back. Feet hip-width apart or more. Knees can be bent to help lengthen your spine. It's fine if heels do not touch the floor.

19. Repeat 11–18, other side

20. Standing forward fold

21. Mountain pose

Repeat sequence 11–18, other side.

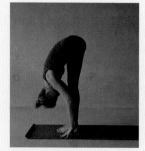
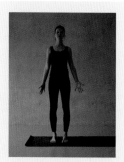

Fold from the hips. Bend knees if necessary.

Standing tall, press down into four corners of feet. Squeeze thighs towards each other. Hands by your sides extending through fingers.

For the following sequence 22–28: do sequence on one side with right leg standing (lifting left leg) and then the other side (with left leg standing and right lifting) as indicated below.

22. Standing quad stretch

…could save those that crossed his path.

23. High lunge with arms clasped behind back

24. Plank

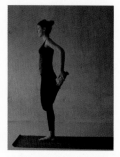
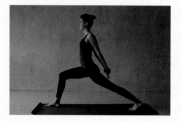
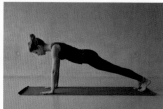

Keep knees close to each other. Then step back with lifted foot into next position.

Ensure that the front knee does not collapse inwards towards the body's midline. Draw shoulders down.

Core tight. Can have knees on floor in a half plank.

25. Sphinx

One day a frog stood in the
middle of the path.

26. Half frog

27. Downward dog

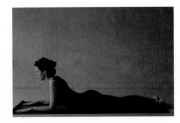

Hips on floor, arms at right angle, core tight, open chest.

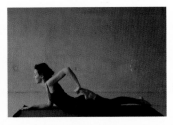

From sphinx, take one foot, pressing it down towards your thigh.

Both sides

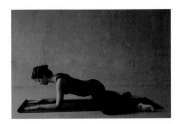

Press hips up and back. Feet hip-width apart or more. Knees can be bent to help lengthen your spine. It's fine if heels do not touch the floor.

'Why do you not cower?' asked
the cobra.

28. Standing forward fold

'Why should I?' asked the frog.

29. Repeat 21–28, other side

30. Sun salutation A with after cobra, wide frog

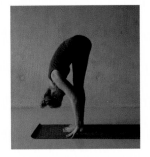

Fold from the hips. Bend knees if necessary.

Repeat sequence 21–28, other side.

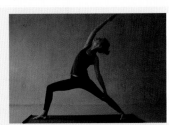

Sun A

See sun salutations.
For wide frog:
from cobra, bring your arms forward to rest on your forearms, widen knees to the side and move hips backwards.

'Because I am fearsome,' the
cobra replied. 'My venom can
injure any warrior who strides in
this forest.'

31. Sun salutation B with after warrior I, warrior II and warrior reverse

Sun B

See sun salutations.

From warrior I,
open into warrior II (see next box).

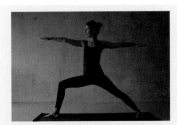

Ensure that your front knee is tracking second toe.

On your inhale, bend back into reverse warrior.

Yoga Fables

For the following sequence 32–37: do the whole sequence on one side first stepping left leg back in 32. From 37, do the other side (stepping right leg back) as indicated below at 38.

The strength of my supple body…

32. Pyramid (with reverse prayer)

…can break the neck of a swan.'

33. Swan

34. Lunge runner's

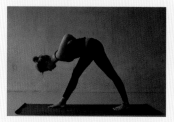
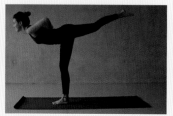
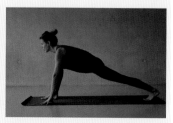

Ensure that hips are level. Can leave front knee slightly bent. For arms in reverse prayer, palms together behind back or just crossed behind, holding elbows.

Either with hands in reverse prayer as shown or hands on floor. Core held tight.

Press into back heel to lengthen.

35. Downward dog (or vinyasa to downward dog)

36. Standing forward fold

37. Mountain pose

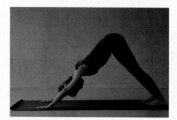
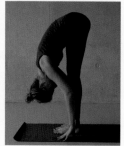
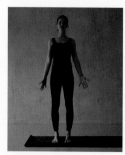

Press hips up and back. Feet hip-width apart or more. Knees can be bent to help lengthen your spine. It's fine if heels do not touch the floor. (See Sun salutation for vinyasa.)

Fold from the hips. Bend knees if necessary.

Standing tall, press down into four corners of feet. Squeeze thighs towards each other. Hands by your sides extending through fingers.

38. Repeat 32–35, other side

39. Plank

'Well,' replied the frog, …

    40. Frog or half frog on both sides

Repeat sequence 32–35, other side.

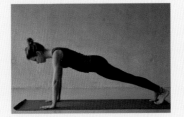

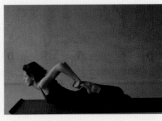

Core tight. Can have knees on floor for half plank.

Press hips down and keep chest open and lifted. Half frog is much easier than frog. For full frog, both legs are held back.

'I have hopped away from arrows from the boys' bows.'

    41. Bow

The cobra snorted. 'My mouth can engulf an entire child!'

    42. Child pose

'Maybe you are mighty; but only until you meet those that are mightier than you,' retorted the frog.

    43. Downward dog

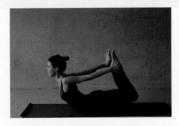

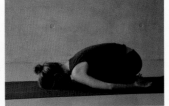

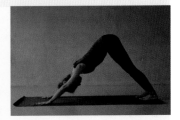

Draw belly button in. Press feet into hands and lengthen front of body.

If your head does not reach the floor, you can place it on your stacked hands or fists.

Press hips up and back. Feet hip-width apart or more. Knees can be bent to help lengthen your spine. It's fine if heels do not touch the floor.

The pigeon swooped down on the cobra's head, momentarily blinding him.

    44. Pigeon

    45. Downward dog

    46. Repeat 44–45, other side

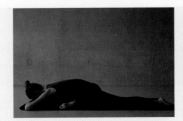

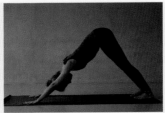

Repeat sequence 44–45, other side.

Ensure that hips are level. Can have a cushion or block under buttock of bent knee. If front knee is uncomfortable, do 'eye of needle pose' instead (see posture index).

Press hips up and back. Feet hip-width apart or more. Knees can be bent to help lengthen your spine. It's fine if heels do not touch the floor.

The king lion roared…

47. Lion

…and swiped the cobra from the side.

48. Bharadvaja's twist

He flew into the air, twisting…

49. Revolved gate

…and tumbling…

50. Repeat 48–49, other side
51. Seated forward fold

…before landing outstretched on the ground.

52. Relaxation pose

Hopping back to his pond, the frog called back to the stricken cobra, 'I at least know that I am just a frog.'

53. Supine extended twist

The cobra reflected on himself, mulling over the frog's words. Maybe he was no more or less than anyone else.

54. Legs up the wall

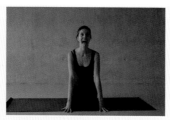

Sit back on heels, stick your tongue out and roar.

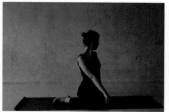

Sitting with both feet pointing to one side, ensure that hips are level. Sit one buttock on cushion if necessary to level hips. Keep spine tall as you twist away from your feet.

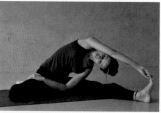

Keep both sit bones grounded and side ribs facing the sky. If bent knee uncomfortable with foot pointing backwards, do 'revolved head to knee' pose instead (see posture index).

Repeat sequence 48–49, other side.

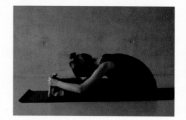

Keep both sit bones grounded. Fold from the hips. Can bend the knees if lower back is uncomfortable.

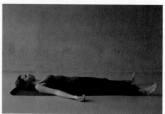

Can have knees bent.

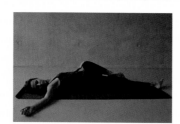

Keep both shoulders on floor. Both sides

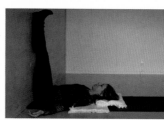

The Warrior and the Eagle

'To be yourself in a world that is constantly trying to make you something
else is the greatest accomplishment.'

Ralph Waldo Emerson

'We discover ourselves when we are faced with an obstacle.'

Saint-Exupéry

Salem was a strong warrior, the highest-ranking warrior in all of the nearby villages. His strength was unmatched. Many came from far away to watch Salem train and fight. His prowess brought him riches, and therefore a comfortable life, along with fame. Yet, despite his successes, despite living a comfortable life, Salem was deeply unhappy. He always wanted to be a better warrior, a stronger human being.

One day while undertaking his usual training, he saw a large eagle swoop and catch his prey. There was such grace and power in this animal. Salem immediately desired to be like that eagle. And so he trained harder, trying to imitate the eagle's flight. His awe for the eagle grew as he tried to personify this king of the sky. Each night, he prayed to embody the eagle's grace and strength. Although his training brought him nearer to his goal, each night doubts and fear of failing plagued his sleep.

Word of the warrior's quest to embody an eagle spread; and soon a crowd joined the usual fans to watch the warrior train. The crowd gasped in awe at his strength and grace. Swelling with pride, the warrior leapt into the flight of the eagle.

All sound was suspended for a moment as the warrior leapt into the air. Then laughter exploded like ripples on a still lake. 'He looks more like a crow than an eagle,' a jarring voice rang out. The mirth continued and the warrior froze, shame-faced.

As the crowds dispersed, the warrior sank to the floor, his heart breaking as his worst fears manifested. He had failed and was humiliated. In this moment of rock-bottom despair, he drew himself deep into his soul. All the fear and doubt that had followed him all his life as a warrior slowly crept over him like ice tentacles searing his heart.

His eyes caught a flicker from the side. In the field next to him was a herd of cows. Salem, still numb with pain, slowly went over to the field, a faraway smile of familiarity reaching the corners of his mouth. As a young boy, Salem had spent much time helping his best friend tend to the cows. It was a time he had loved and which had planted a seed of desire in his heart. A seed he had shunned and shut away because his family and he himself had wanted a life better than that of a mere cow herder. He was to be a warrior. But not just any warrior! He had sought to be the best warrior there ever was. Yet even that had not been enough; he needed to be like the king of the sky — an eagle.

Salem laughed. He was not an eagle. He was not even truly a warrior. He was a man who had enjoyed looking after the cows. He was a man called Salem. He was himself and that was enough. Breathing deeply for the first time, he found his way home.

Sequence: The Warrior and the Eagle

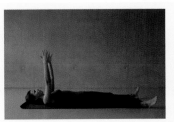 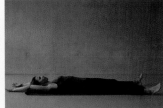 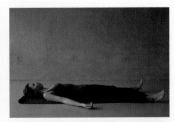

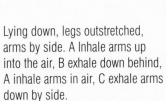 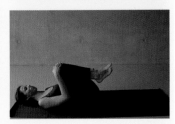

Lying down, legs outstretched, arms by side. A Inhale arms up into the air, B exhale down behind, A inhale arms in air, C exhale arms down by side.
Repeat.

2 times

Keep extended leg pressing down and core tight as you bring forehead to knee.

Both sides

With both knees to chest, widen knees apart and then bring them back together in a circular motion. Change direction.

3 times

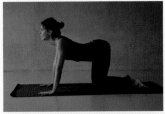 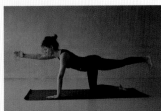 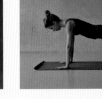

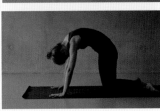

Inhale on A and exhale on B.

3-6 times

Extend one leg and opposite arm, keeping your core tight.
2 times each side

Keep core tight. Can be on knees for a half plank.

7. Push-ups

…yet unhappy…

8. Child pose

…because he thinks he needs to be stronger…

9. Downward dog

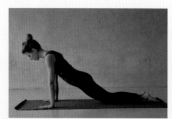

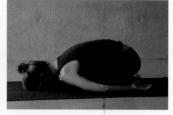

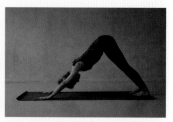

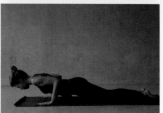

↑ If your head does not reach the floor, you can place it on your stacked hands or fists.
← Can have knees off the floor. Core tight. Two arm positions: a) elbows close to ribs (as shown), b) elbows out wide. Press to straighten and bend arms in push-ups. 3 times each position

Press hips up and back. Feet hip-width apart or more. Knees can be bent to help lengthen your spine. It's fine if heels do not touch the floor.

…and better.

10. Downward dog split
11. Crescent moon lunge
12. Repeat 9–11, other side

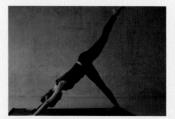

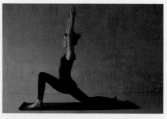

Repeat sequence 9–11 on other side.

From downward dog, lift one leg up. Place lifted leg forward into next pose.

Ensure that the front knee does not collapse inwards towards the body's midline.

13. Downward dog

14. Standing forward fold

One day, while undertaking his usual training…

15. Sun salutations A

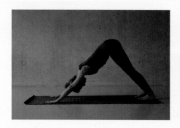

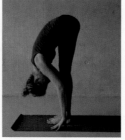

Sun A

Press hips up and back. Feet hip-width apart or more. Knees can be bent to help lengthen your spine. It's fine if heels do not touch the floor.

Fold from the hips. Bend knees if necessary.

See sun salutations.
(Can add knee crunches, bringing knee forward and rounding spine from downward dog).
2 times

16. Fierce pose or Sun B

…he sees an eagle.

17. Eagle

He starts to train harder…

18. Sun B with after warrior I, pyramid pose and warrior III

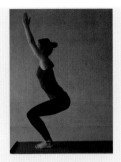

See sun salutations.
Feet and knees together, sit back, keeping spine long.

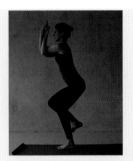

Right leg on top with left arm on top (cross at elbows and touch palms. A modifiction closer to full pose but quite achievable is instead backs of hands together, rather than palms).
If cannot wind foot around calf, can just have legs crossed.
Can also leave top foot grounded.

Both sides

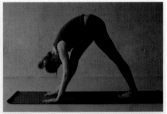

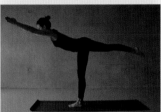

See sun salutations. From warrior I, step back foot forward a little and straighten front knee, fold over for pyramid pose. Ensure hips are even. From here take weight onto front foot, lifting the back into warrior III. Keep core tight.

19. Mountain pose

20. Fierce pose

…to be like the eagle.

21. Eagle pose

For the following sequence 19 to 28: Do sequence on one side and then the other to 27 as indicated below.

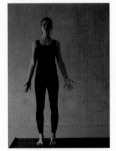

Standing tall, press down into four corners of feet. Squeeze thighs towards each other. Hands by your sides extending through fingers.

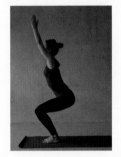

Feet and knees together, sit back, keeping spine long.

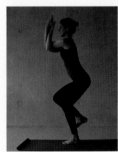

1st time right leg on top with left arm on top. 2nd time left leg on top with right arm on top. Unwind top leg and hinge into next pose.

22. Eagle warrior III

His awe grows…
23. Warrior I

…and he prays to embody the eagle's strength.
24. Humble warrior

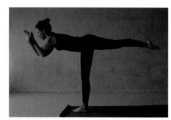

Keep both hips level and core held tight.

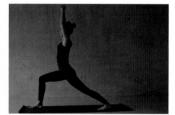

Ensure that knee does not collapse inwards towards the body's midline. Your hips and torso are facing the front of your mat.

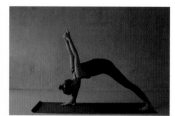

From warrior I, fold from the hips with hands clasped behind, arms lifting off your back.

25. Lunge runner's

26. Vinyasa to downward dog

Yet each night doubts plague him.
27. Child pose extended

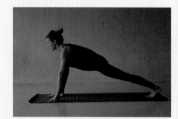

Press into back heel to lengthen.

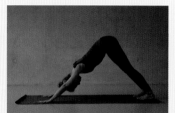

See sun salutations

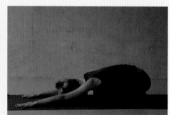

Sitting back on your heels, lengthen your arms in front.

28. Standing forward fold

Word of the warrior's quest to embody an eagle spreads and a crowd join to watch the warrior train.

The crowd gasp at his strength.
29. Repeat 19–27, other side

30. Boat

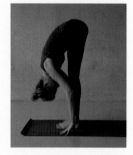

Fold from the hips. Bend knees if necessary.

Repeat 19–27, other side.

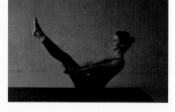

Keep back straight with core held tight. Can have knees bent.

The warrior swells with pride.

31. Cat–cow

32. Downward dog (with crunches)

He leaps into the air…

33. Squat

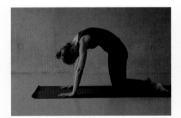

Inhale on A, exhale on B.

3 times

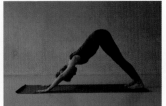

From downward dog position, bring one knee towards front of mat and then lift leg up behind. Change sides.
3 times

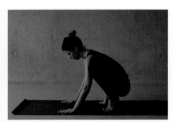

Bring knees above elbows and squeeze thighs.

…but only manages to look like a crow to the laughing crowd.

34. Crow

The warrior freezes, shamefaced, sinking to the ground in despair.

35. Child pose

He draws himself deep into his soul.

36. Half lord of the fishes

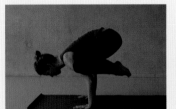

Looking forward, knees above elbows, squeeze thighs and lift feet off the ground through drawing in pelvic floor. Can lift just one foot, then the other.

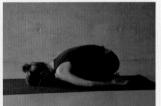

If your head does not reach the floor, you can place it on your stacked hands or fists.

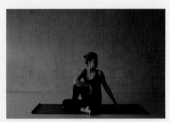

Can leave bottom leg straight instead of folded back. Root into sit bones, and keep spine long as you twist towards your bent knee.

He sees the cows in the next field.

37. Cow-face pose

38. Repeat 36–37, other side

And remembers his youth and fondness for cow herding. He remembers how he had tried to be what others expected;

39. Staff pose

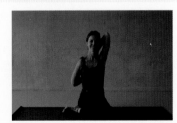

Can have bottom leg extended. Clasp hands behind back or clasp a belt.

Repeat sequence 36–37, on other side.

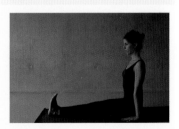

Keep both sit bones grounded and spine tall.

...to be what he thought was more important.

40. Bridge

41. Knees to chest

He realises that he is not what he tried to be...

42. (Half) shoulder stand

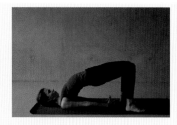

With feet parallel, lift hips up keeping knees in line with your hips. You can clasp your hands behind back.

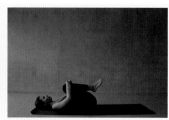

Press hips into the floor to lengthen the spine.

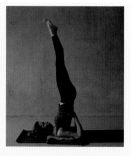

Have arms and shoulders on a blanket to protect the neck.
also do half shoulder stand, Can where legs are angled slightly over head to make body into a C-shape.

...and that being himself is enough.

43. Plough

He breathes deeply for the first time.

44. Fish

45. Supine twist

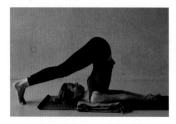

Can have shoulders supported by a blanket as shown to stress the neck less.

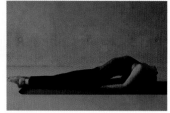

Hands under buttocks with palms on the mat. Elbows tight against ribcage. Lift on to elbows and arch back and neck, gently resting head on the mat.

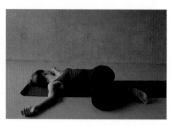

Keep both shoulders on the floor.

Both sides

And goes home.

46. Supine knees to chest

47. Relaxation

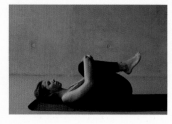

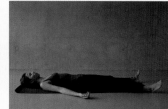

Can also have knees bent.

The Silence of Snow

'Peace comes from within. Do not seek it without.'

Buddha

'Learning how to be still, to really be still and let life happen – that stillness becomes radiance.'

Morgan Freeman

In the grey twilight, soft flakes drifted down to blanket the earth. The black cat stretched atop the shallow bridge to watch the cold white feathers as they gently swirled, danced and levitated down. The landscape dulled to shades of white and shadow. Crispness moistened the cat's whiskers and nose as it welcomed the snow. Its fur glistened like black velvet studded with opals. A hush as deep as a breath in the pearly landscape, sound muted, could be heard from the mountain brook below.

The cat settled atop the bridge, content in winter's gift, its fur warm beneath a settling white blanket. Its ears perked to one side then the other, listening, hearing, the silence brought by the settled snow. Far away were busy minds; far away was activity rife; far away were those who knew not the quiet peace of the snow. Curled up on the bridge, the cat rested peaceful and protected by the white. Nothing interrupted its deep rest, its breath in concert with the falling snowflakes. The world fell quiet as stars appeared in the sky and as the moonlight, shimmering, awoke a thousand stars across the countryside. Out of the silence of the snow the cat stirred to play refreshed in the pearl landscape below.

Sequence: The Silence of Snow

Equipment: 1–2 bolsters (or large pillows or piles of blankets), 3 blankets, 1 pillow, 2 blocks.
You can be inventive with the equipment. Keep the overall shape of the pose but adjust for comfort.
This is a restorative yoga sequence. After the 'warm-up' (1), make yourself as comfortable as possible and lie in each pose for 5–15min.

A black cat stretched…

1. Cat–cow

…atop a shallow bridge to watch the cold white feathers as they gently swirled, danced and levitated down.

2. Supported bridge

A hush as deep as a breath is heard from the mountain brook below.

3. Mountain brook

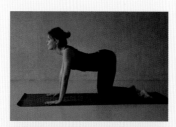

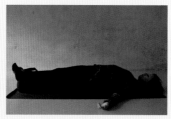

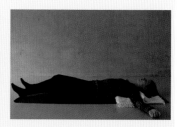

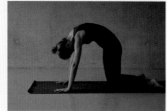

Inhale on A and exhale on B.

3-6 times

Use two bolsters if possible. Top bolster ends at mid back. Shoulders are on floor or blanket(s), head supported. A strap can be placed on feet to hold them together.
Or can have one block under the sacrum and knees bent.
Can have pillow or blanket under shoulders, head.

One blanket under upper back (shoulders on floor, not on blanket) and one for head. Bolster supporting knees.

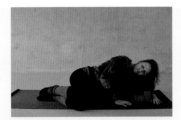

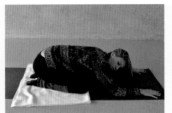

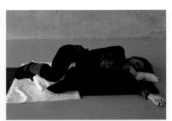

The cat settled atop the bridge, content in winter's gift, its fur warm beneath a settling white blanket. Its ears perked to one side then the other, listening, hearing, the silence brought by the settled snow.

4. Elevated side and twist

Curled up on the bridge, the cat rested peaceful and protected by the white.

5. Child pose

Nothing interrupted its deep rest, its breath in concert with the falling snowflakes.

6. Side-lying or supported relaxation

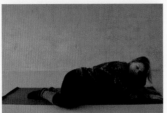

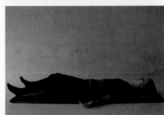

Lie for a couple of minutes on side on an elevated bolster (one end on a few blocks), with head supported by cushion or a folded blanket. Then twist from lower belly on to bolster. Head can stay on same side or twist to other if comfortable with neck.
One side, then the other.
Moving slowly to transition.

Legs wide, seated on heels, torso on bolster. Change head to other side halfway through.

Lie on side, head on a blanket or pillow, with a blanket between the knees. Top arm is supported by the bolster.Or lie on back with knees supported by bolster.

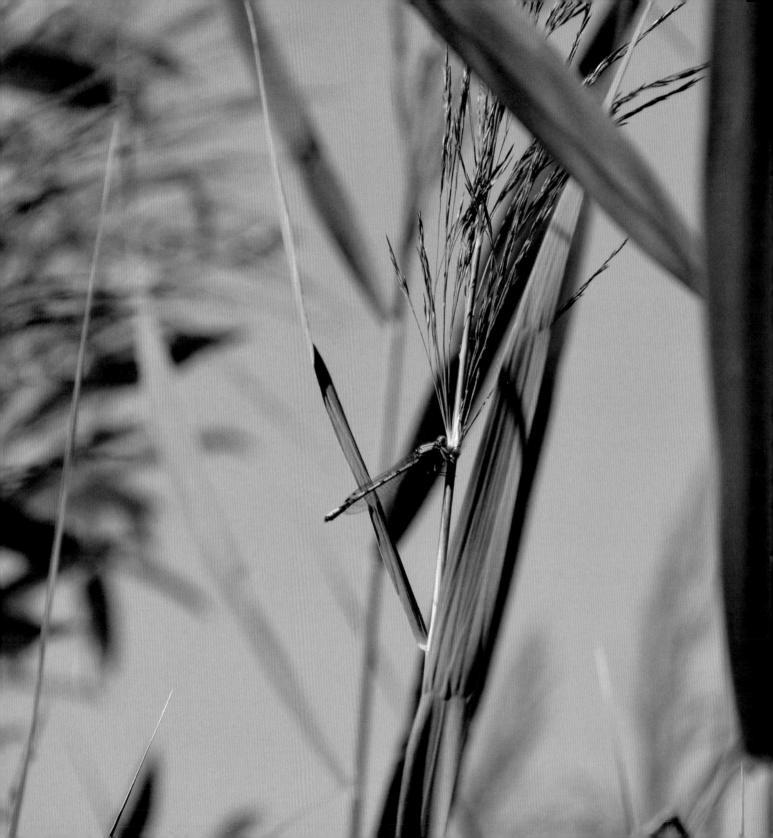

The Lord of the Sky

'Don't cry because it's over, smile because it happened.'

Dr Seuss

'Happiness is a journey, not a destination; happiness is to be found along the way not at the end of the road, for then the journey is over and it's too late.'

Paul Harold Dunn

In a secluded glade by the waterfall, Xsariana played among the rock pools, waiting for her fishing nets to catch her family's supper. She delighted in the rainbows of the spray, the fuchsia flowers among the lush green and the deep blue of the pool beneath her.

A glitter from above made her stand still as rock, like a deer that had seen its hunter. High above at the top of the waterfall stood a man with golden hair fluttering in the wind; not a man, a warrior; not a warrior, a god. From where she was, she could see a smile, but she still stood frozen as fear was replaced by fascination, by awe and by the first flutters of her heart. He began a slow but deliberate dance that seemed to Xsariana like a courting dance. Her heart melted at the sight and soon she found her body responding in kind. She was in love.

The god stood graceful like a warrior and bowed to her. And then as he started to launch himself off the waterfall towards her, his arms spread into wings; and soon a large eagle flew to a branch above her. Xsariana gazed up at the Lord of the Sky. She brought out her flute and played for him. The melancholy tune was full of the hope of love. She played oblivious to the passing hours, to the changing hue of the sky. As the sun started to set the eagle looked up and expanded his wings to fly. Fearful of the coming loss, Xsariana started to dance, willing the Lord of the Sky to stay with her. He hesitated for a heartbeat before inevitably answering the call of the sky.

Looking toward the sky and the first stars appearing, Xsariana offered her heart. Not accepting nature's way, she tried every way to communicate to the gods her love for the Lord of the Sky. But she was a woman of the earth, not a creature of the sky, nor a goddess.

A chime brought her out of her obsessive thoughts. The bell on her nets notified her that she had caught fish. As she went to gather her bounty, she looked deep within the dark pool reflecting not only the approaching night but also the darkness of her thoughts. She had been swept away by her passions for that which she could not keep, that which she could not own. As one cannot keep the day from turning into night, so she could not keep the Lord of the Sky.

The moon rose to light the sky and in the pool she saw the reflection of an eagle flying high. Looking up, a smile lit her eyes. Caught up in her own passions and feelings of loss, she had disregarded the wonder and blessings that she had been favoured by the Lord of the Sky and that she had shared herself with him. Both had been touched by the magic and that moment was all that was needed.

Sequence: The Lord of the Sky

In a secluded glade...

1. Supine breathing

2. Supine head to knee

3. Hip mobilisation

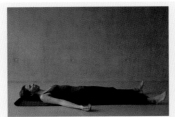

Lying comfortably. Breathe in three parts: belly, ribcage and collarbone.

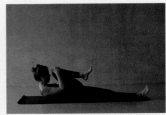

Keep extended leg pressing down and core tight as you bring forehead to knee.

Both sides

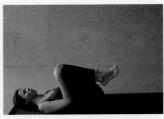

With both knees to chest, widen knees apart and then bring them back together in a circular motion. Change direction.
3 times each direction

4. Eye of needle

5. Supine twist

...Xsariana played among the rock pools.

6. Cat–cow

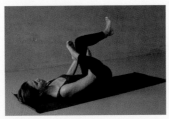

The feet should be flexed and hips on the floor.

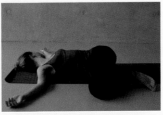

Keep both shoulders on the floor.

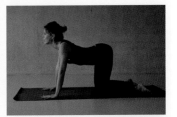

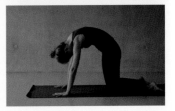

Inhale on A and exhale on B

Both sides

Both sides

3–6 times

7. Dynamic cat

8. Alternate arms and legs

9. Downward dog

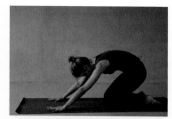

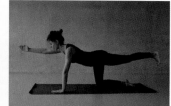

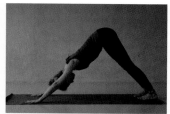

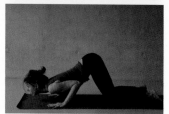

↑ Extend one leg and opposite arm, keeping your core tight. Both sides

← Starting on all fours, A exhale, rounding back and sitting on heels, B inhale, sweeping forward chin towards floor, coming back to all fours. Repeat. 3–6 times

Press hips up and back. Feet hip-width apart or more. Knees can be bent to help lengthen your spine. It's fine if heels do not touch the floor.

10. Crescent moon lunge

11. Low lunge prayer twist

12. Downward dog

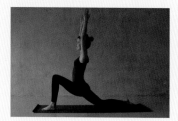

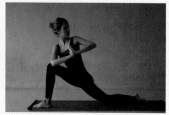

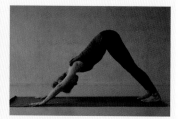

Ensure that the front knee does not collapse inwards towards the body's midline.

Keep chest open as you twist placing your elbow on knee.

13. Repeat 10–12 on the other side

14. Standing forward fold

High above at the top of the waterfall stood a man…no…

15. Standing prayer

Repeat sequence 10–12, other side.

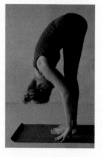

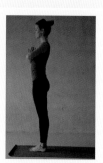

Fold from the hips. Bend knees if necessary.

Standing tall, press down into four corners of feet. Squeeze thighs towards each other. Palms together at heart centre.

…a god.

16. Reach the sky

He began a slow but deliberate dance…

17. Fierce pose

18. Albatross

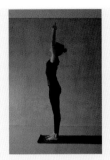

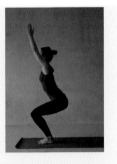

Feet and knees together, sit back, keeping spine long.

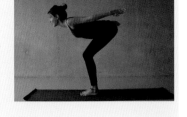

From fierce pose, hinge at hips with a straight back, core tight.

19. Standing forward fold arms behind

20. Downward dog split

21. Standing forward fold

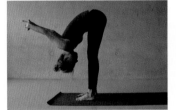

Fold from the hips. Bend knees if necessary. The arms may not lift much from back.

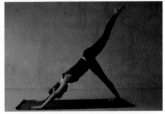

From downward dog, lift one leg up.

Both sides

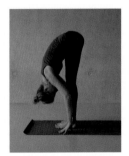

22. Mountain pose

23. Standing hand to foot & side

24. Eagle prep

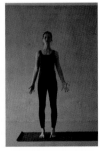

Standing tall, press down into four corners of feet. Squeeze thighs towards each other. Hands by your sides extending through fingers.

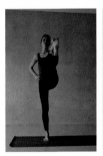

To keep back straight, can just hold bent knee towards chest instead and then open to the side.

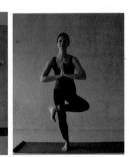

Bend standing leg and place lifted ankle on knee, sitting further in pose.

25. Repeat 22–24, other side

26. Standing prayer

Xsariana found her body responding in kind.

27. Sun salutation A or Classical sun salutation

Repeat sequence 22–24, other side.

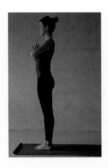

Sun A or Classical sun salutation
See sun salutations.

For the following sequence 28–34: do the whole sequence on one side, stepping left leg back into 28. From 34, step right leg back into 28 as indicated in 35.

Like a warrior he stood graceful…

28. Warrior I

…and bowed to her.

29. Humble warrior

And then as he started to launch himself towards her…

30. High lunge with eagle arms

…his arms spread into wings;

31. (Warrior III with eagle arms) – optional

and soon a large eagle flew to a branch above her.

32. Eagle

Xsariana brought out her flute and played for him.

33. Krishna

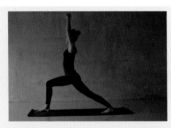

Ensure that knee does not collapse inwards towards the body's midline. Your hips and torso are facing the front of your mat.

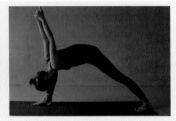

From warrior I, fold from the hips with hands clasped behind, lifting arms off back.

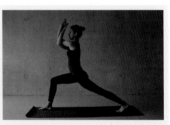

Cross same arm as front leg on top.

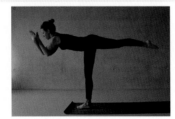

From above position, draw weight on to front leg and bend torso forward, lifting back heel off the floor.

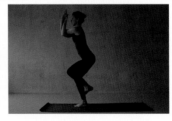

Sweep back leg up and over bent standing leg into pose. Keep standing leg bent.

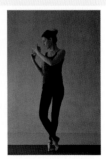

Place toe on floor.
Twist to one side and then the other.

34. Standing side stretches

35. Repeat 28–34, other side

As the sun started to set the eagle looked up and expanded his wings to fly.

36. Classical sun salutation with low lunge quad stretch

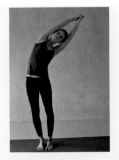

Keep both feet anchored with equal weight as you bend.

Both sides

Repeat sequence 28–34, other side.

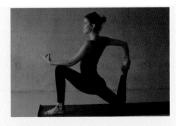

Classical sun salutation with low lunge quad stretch.
See sun salutations. On the low lunge, can grasp back foot in a quad stretch. Omit if not comfortable or possible.

Xsariana started to dance, willing the Lord of the Sky to stay with her.

37. Dancer's pose

38. Standing forward fold

He hesitated a heartbeat before answering the call of the sky.

39. Kneeling with lotus mudra

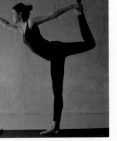

Keep both hips pointing forward.

Both sides

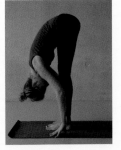

Fold from hips. Can have knees bent.

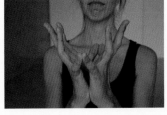

Sit on heels. Heel of hands, little fingers and thumbs together. Ten full breaths.

Looking toward the sky, Xsariana offered her heart.

40. Bridge

41. Wheel – optional

42. Supine knees to chest

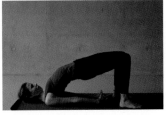

With feet parallel, lift hips up keeping knees in line with your hips. You can clasp your hands behind back.

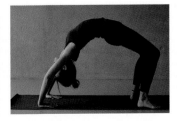

From bridge, place hands behind head, lift up on to head, then push arms straight. Come down as you came up.

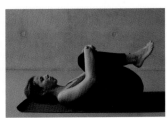

Press hips into the floor to lengthen the spine.

She tried every way to communicate to the gods her love.

43. Supine twist

44. (Half) shoulder stand

45. Plough

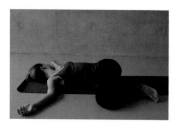

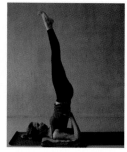

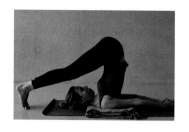

Keep both shoulders on the floor.

Both sides

Have arms and shoulders on a blanket to protect the neck. Can also do half shoulder stand, where legs are angled slightly over head to make body into a C-shape.

Can have shoulders supported by a blanket as shown to stress the neck less.

A chime from her nets notifying her of caught fish brought her out of her obsessive thoughts.

46. Fish

She looked deep within the dark pool.

47. Head to knee pose

48. Revolved head to knee pose

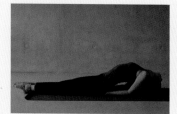

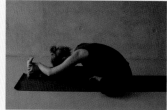

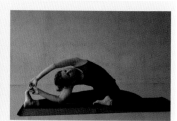

Hands under buttocks with palms on the mat. Elbows tight against ribcage. Lift on to elbows and arch back and neck, gently resting head on the mat.

Keep both sit bones grounded. Fold from the hips over extended leg. Can bend the knee if lower back is uncomfortable.

Keep both sit bones grounded and side ribs facing sky. Can bend the extended leg if necessary.

49. Half lord of the fishes pose

The moon rose high to light the sky and in the pool she saw the reflection of an eagle flying high.

50. Repeat 47–49, other side.

51. Supine knees to chest

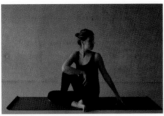

Repeat sequence 47–49, other side.

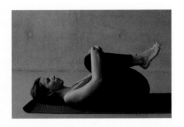

Can leave bottom leg straight instead of folded back. Root into sit bones, and keep spine long as you twist towards your bent knee.

Press hips into the floor to lengthen the spine.

Looking up, she smiled. Both had been touched by the magic…

52. Supine butterfly pose

…and that moment was all that was needed.

53. Relaxation

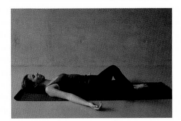

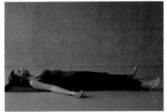

Feet together with knees opening to the side.

Can have knees bent.

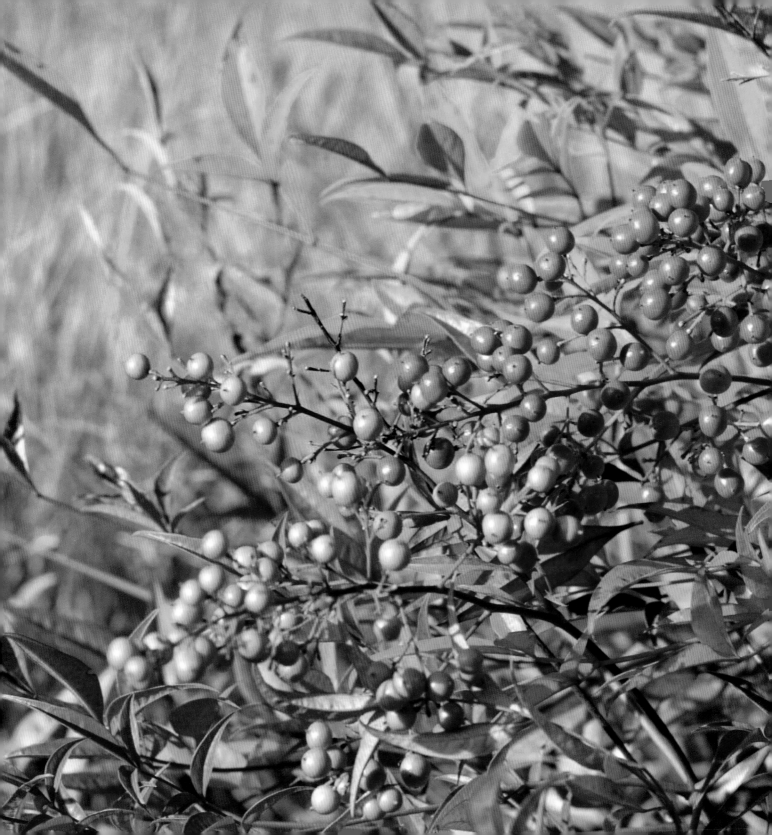

Mother Dog

'You cannot serve from an empty vessel. When you take time to replenish your spirit,
it allows you to serve others from the overflow.'

Eleanor Brownn

'You yourself, as much as anybody in the entire universe, deserve your love and affection.'

Buddha

Mother Dog sat at the corner of the fence, her watchful eyes surveying the prairie. The speckled cat was stretching in the morning sun; her own pup trying to imitate the cat. Mother Dog rose to urge her pup to go eat his breakfast. The pup jumped around playfully while Mother Dog shooed him back towards the farm, warning him he should take care of himself and eat his breakfast. The pup sank down in front of his bowl, shamefaced.

The farmer came out of the building, carrying his scythe to cut some hay. Mother Dog watched him at his work from under a tree. He was working hard, too hard as usual. Mother Dog ran up to him barking that he should take it easier, that he should take care of himself.

The farmer's son ran into the yard, a toy sword in his hand. He shouted with glee as he fenced, hit, ran and jumped; and finally tripped and fell. Mother Dog ran up to him, licking his face, and told him to take better care of himself.

Close by, Mother Dog's prairie friends Grass Snake, Grasshopper and Toad were all out foraging for food. She ran up to them to warn them of the farmer who was *nearby cutting hay. They should take more care, she urged, worry in her voice. Wood Pigeon flapped by being lazily chased by the farmer's boy. Mother Dog barked to the pigeon to take care of itself.*

The sun beating down, Mother Dog sat, her ears twitching worriedly, her tongue panting, as she surveyed the farm and her 'children'. She tried her best to take care of them all but they still seemed to get into trouble.

Tiredness swept through Mother Dog as the sun went down. She sank down, worry still on her brow, surveying the farm. Everyone seemed happy enough though. She curled up, feeling exhaustedly content that she had looked after everyone today. As her lids closed it occurred to her that she had neither drunk nor eaten. But that did not matter to her because she had looked after them all. Tomorrow she would do the same. But tomorrow almost never came for Mother Dog, who had taken care of all but herself.

A warm gust of air, a cold nose against her own; a whimper in her ear; a caress; a soft voice in her head telling her she was loved, that she deserved to take care of herself. She took an inspired breath of fresh air with a resolve that she would.

Sequence: Mother Dog

Mother Dog surveys the prairie...

1. Seated neck stretches
2. Seated side stretch
3. Seated twist

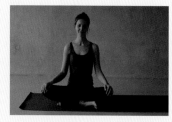

In a comfortable seated position, turn head side to side and then move on to some neck rolls.

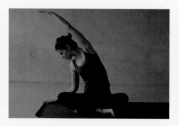

Keep both sit bones grounded and side ribs facing the sky as you bend.

Both sides

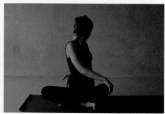

Keep both sit bones grounded and chest open as you twist.

Both sides

The cat stretches in the sunlight.

4. Cat–cow

The puppy is trying to imitate the cat.

5. Dynamic cat

6. Puppy

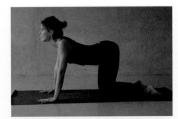 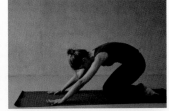 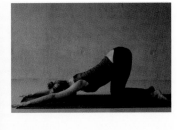

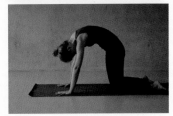 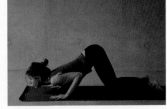

Inhale on A and exhale on B

Starting on all fours, A exhale, rounding back and sitting on heels, B inhale, sweeping forward chin towards floor, coming back to all fours. Repeat.

Hips lifted, lengthen spine with arms reaching forward.

3–6 times

3–6 times

Mother Dog shoos the puppy…

7. Downward dog

…who is jumping around playfully.

8. Downward dog split

9. Crescent moon lunge

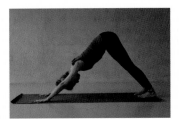 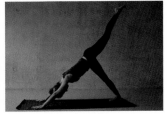 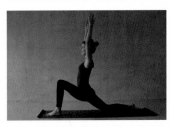

Press hips up and back. Feet hip-width apart or more. Knees can be bent to help lengthen your spine. It's fine if heels do not touch the floor.

From downward dog, lift one leg up.

Place lifted foot forward into lunge. Ensure that the front knee does not collapse inwards towards the body's midline.

She tells him to take care of himself.

| 10. Repeat 7–9, other side |
| 11. Downward dog |
| 12. Plank |

Repeat sequence 7–9, other side.

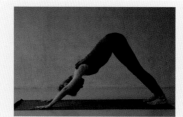

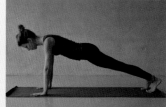

Core held tight. Can have knees on floor.

The puppy sinks shamefaced towards his bowl.

| 13. Sphinx |
| 14. Downward dog |
| 15. Standing forward fold |

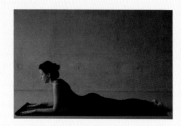

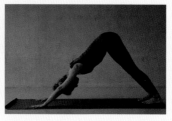

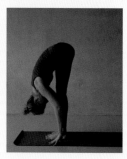

Hips on floor, arms at right angle, core tight, open chest.

Press hips up and back. Feet hip-width apart or more. Knees can be bent to help lengthen your spine. It's fine if heels do not touch the floor.

Step both feet forward into pose.

The farmer comes out to do his work…

| 16. Mountain pose |
| 17. Reach the sky |
| 18. Squat |

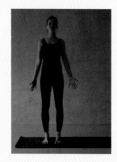

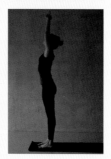

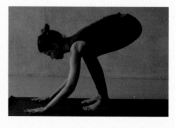

Standing tall, press down into four corners of feet. Squeeze thighs towards each other. Hands by your sides extending through fingers.

Bend knees to touch floor and then sweep up to standing arms over head to next pose.

19. Standing side bends

20. Standing forward fold

21. Standing twist

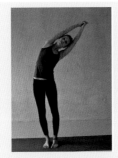

Keep both feet anchored with equal weight as you bend.

Both sides; 2 times

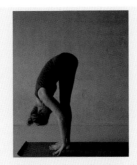

Fold from hips. Can have knees bent.

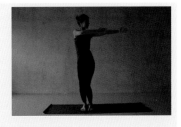

Keep both feet anchored with equal weight as you twist.

Both sides; 2 times

For the following sequence 23–34, do the whole sequence on one side. Then do the other side as indicated in 35.

22. Reach the sky, then hands prayer

...carrying his scythe to cut some hay.

23. Standing hand to foot in front and to side

Mother Dog sits under the tree and watches...

24. Tree

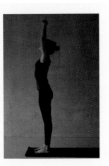

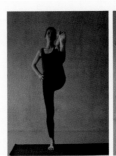

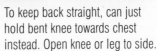

To keep back straight, can just hold bent knee towards chest instead. Open knee or leg to side.

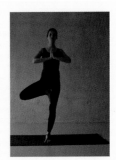

Can either rest lifted foot on floor near ankle, on shin or on thigh (not on knee). Can also lift hands overhead. Step lifted leg back into next pose.

...the hard work of the farmer.

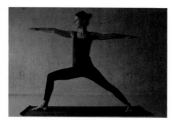 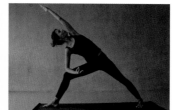 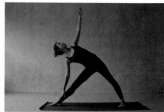

Ensure that knee does not go over ankle and is tracking second toe. Torso is open to the side.

Keep weight even on both feet. Can also place hand on floor inside the leg, if possible, instead of having elbow on the thigh.

From side angle pose, straighten front knee. Can have top arm on hip rather than extended.

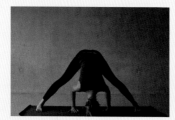 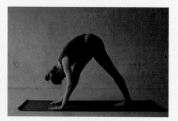 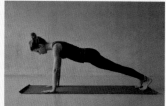

Feet wide, turned very slightly inward. Fold from hips. Can have knees (slightly) bent.

Turn towards front of mat, stepping back foot in a little. Keep hips square as you fold over.

Core tight.

Mother Dog runs up to tell him to take care of himself.

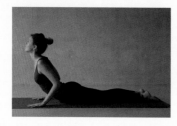 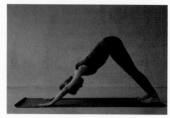 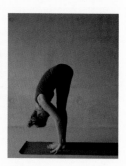

Keep lower back long by pressing pubic bone to floor and keeping core tight. Keep all toenails pressing into ground and open upper chest with elbows close to ribcage.

Press hips up and back. Feet hip-width apart or more. Knees can be bent to help lengthen your spine. It's fine if heels do not touch the floor.

Step feet to front of mat.

34. Mountain pose

35. Repeat 23–34, other side

*The farmer's boy runs into the
yard playing.*

36. Sun salutation B

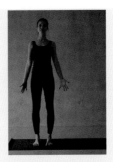

Repeat sequence 23–34,
other side.

Standing tall, press down into four
corners of feet. Squeeze thighs
towards each other. Hands by your
sides extending through fingers.

Sun B

See sun salutations.
After final downward dog come
into child's pose as follows.

He trips and falls.

37. Child pose

*Mother Dog runs up to tell him to
take care of himself.*

38. Downward dog

39. Plank

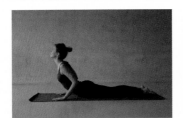

If your head does not reach the floor,
you can place it on your stacked
hands or fists.

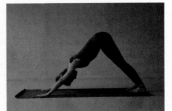

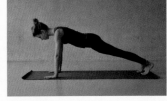

Core tight.

Her friends, Grass Snake…

40. Cobra

…Grasshopper and…

41. Locust

…Toad are foraging nearby.

42. Half frog

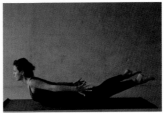

Keep lower back long by pressing
pubic bone to floor and keeping
core tight. Keep all toenails pressing
into the ground and open upper
chest with elbows close to ribcage.

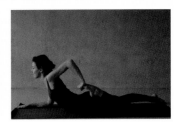

Extend in length rather than height.
Keep hips planted and core tight.
Can also extend arms forward.
Inhale lifting, exhale down.

Keep hips to floor and core tight
coming to rest on forearms. Clasp a
foot and press towards thigh.

Both sides

Mother Dog runs up to tell them to take care of themselves.

43. Downward dog

Wood Pigeon flaps by being chased by the boy.

44. Pigeon

Mother Dog runs up to tell it to take care of itself.

45. Repeat 43–44, other side

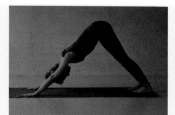

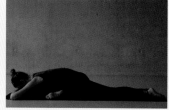

Repeat sequence 43–44, other side.

If hips are not level, place a cushion or block under folded leg buttock. If front knee is uncomfortable, come out of posture and do eye of needle pose instead.

Mother Dog sat…

46. Extended child pose

…her ears twitching worriedly…

47. Kneeling cow-face arms (thunder-bolt with cow-face arms)

…her tongue panting…

48. Lion

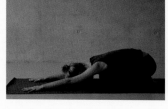

Sit back on heels with arms outstretched.

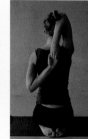

If cannot reach hands, can hold a strap.
Both sides

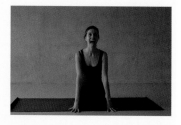

Stick tongue out and exhale loudly.

…as she surveyed the farm and her 'children'.

49. Bharadvaja's twist (or seated twist)

Tired, she sinks down.

50. Seated wide angle forward fold

Everyone seems happy.

51. Happy baby pose

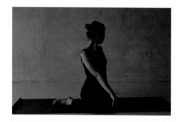

Sitting with both feet pointing to one side, ensure that hips are level. Sit one buttock on cushion if necessary to level hips. Keep spine tall as you twist away from your feet.

Both sides

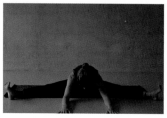

Fold from hips, keeping spine long Then walk hands to one leg.

Both sides.

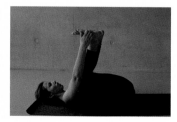

Grasp feet or shins and keep pelvis on floor.

She curled up. She had looked after everyone today – except herself.

52. Supine twist

She sleeps, unable to get up the next day.

53. Relaxation

A soft voice told her she was loved and that she deserved to take care of herself.

54. Meditation

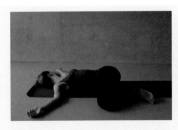

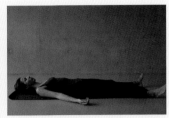

Keep both shoulders on the floor. Both sides

Can have knees bent.

Either supine or seated, focussing on breath in belly, listening to the heartbeat. Follow breath in heart and belly and observe with self-compassion.

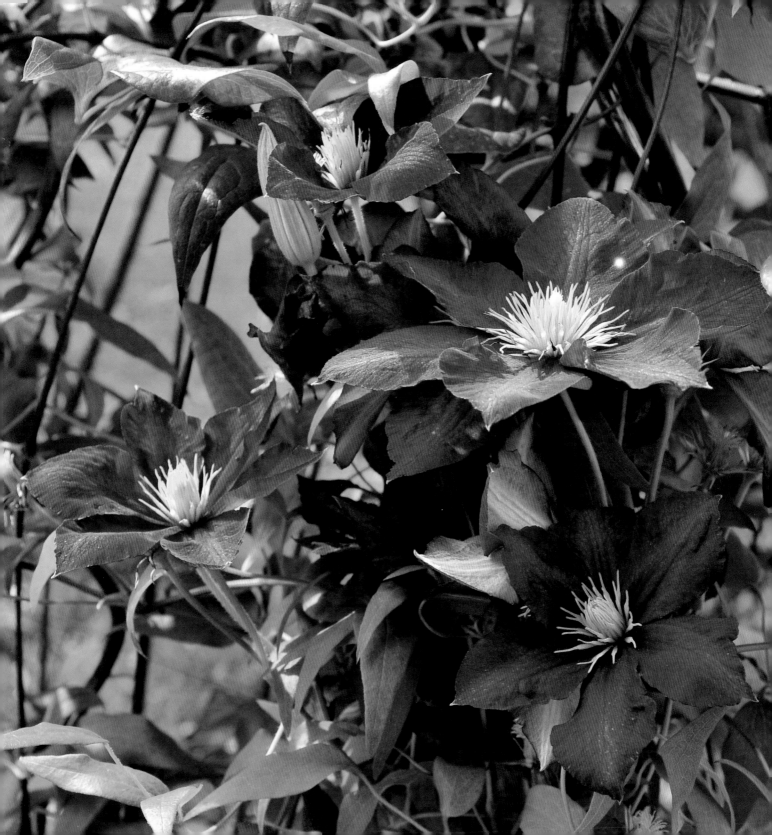

The Mask of the Goddess

'The time has come to turn your heart into a temple of fire. Your essence is gold hidden by dust.
To reveal its splendour you need to burn in the fire of love.'

Rumi

'Over the years, I learned to smile or laugh when I was supposed to. I kept my true self hidden;
I did not need to unleash my pain on the world around me. Instead, I taught myself to ignore it.
I did not realize that the pain was eating away at my soul.'

Joy Stroube

The goddess yawned and stretched. Another day had begun. Another day dedicated to her ritual dance of perfection. She moved lithe as a cat towards her dressing table with its gilded mirror. On it was a beautiful smooth golden mask. With reverence she fixed it upon her face, lifting her gaze to the mirror. Perfection reflected. She smiled. She had to be perfect. She was a goddess after all. The reflection in the mirror seemed to agree with this thought as the brilliance of her mask caught the first rays of the sun.

In her garden, she danced her ritual under the willow tree. She saluted the sky and the earth, concentrating on perfecting her movements. The goddess continued to dance with fluid grace as the first stars appeared in the twilight. Unexpectedly, her poise faltered. Her grace felt disgraced as her dance lost its perfection. Yet she danced on, compelled by a budding desire — for what, she could not yet identify. As her body moved to its own tune, her moon dance became wilder and cracks appeared on her golden mask.

Incandescent in the sky, the moon and stars reflected her flow. Stronger her desire became, like a flame inside her. And she was terrified. A flame wavers and flickers. It had no place in the flawless grace of the goddess that she was. Her heart broke, torn wide open. She no longer knew who she was.

Seated in her temple, her tear-stained gaze fell on the starry night and she prayed. Tuning in to that desire deep inside her, she let her gaze turn inward towards that flickering flame. As she gently let go of who she thought she needed to be, her mask finally broke and she recognised that yearning: it was to be herself. She came face to face with her inner flame, her breath stilled and warmth filled her belly and heart. She knew who she was. She was a goddess; imperfect yet in that instant perfect. She felt an immense joy, a feeling that could only be described as having finally found her way home.

Sequence: The Mask of the Goddess

Will also need 1 bolster, 1 block, 4 blankets and 1 cushion for the restorative poses at the end.

The goddess yawned…
1. Seated side stretch

…and stretched.
2. Seated twist

As lithe as a cat…
3. Cat–cow

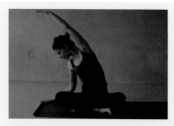

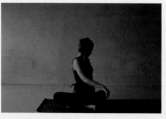

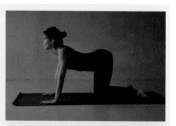

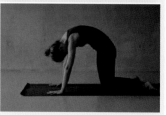

Keep both sit bones grounded and side ribs facing the sky as you bend.

Both sides

↑ Keep both sit bones grounded and chest open as you twist.
Both sides

Inhale on A and exhale on B. →
3–6 times

She moved…

4. Downward dog

…towards her dressing table. On it was a golden mask. With reverence she fixed it…

5. Crescent moon lunge with side bend

…upon her face. In the mirror perfection reflected.

6. Gate pose

She had to be perfect, after all.

7. Kneeling half moon

8. Repeat 4–7 on other side

9. Downward dog

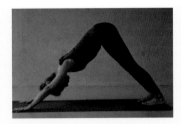

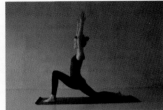

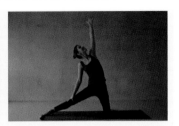

Press hips up and back. Feet hip-width apart or more. Knees can be bent to help lengthen your spine. It's fine if heels do not touch the floor.

Place one foot at front of mat and back knee on floor. Lift arms and side-bend towards the front leg.

Keep hips facing front. Flex sideways over extended leg. Can have the foot of the extended leg flexed (toes up) instead of toes towards the floor.

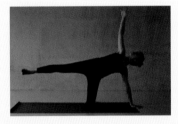

Repeat sequence 4–7, other side.

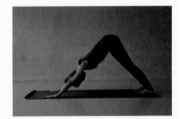

Push through the flexed foot of the extended leg.

For the following sequence 10–18, do the whole sequence on one side. Then do the other as indicated in 19.

10. Standing forward fold

She was a goddess.

11. Reach to sky

She danced her ritual…

12. Shiva Dancing

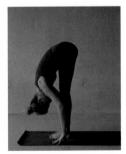

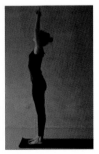

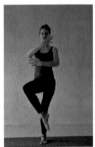

Walk both feet to front of mat.

Standing tall, press down into four corners of feet. Squeeze thighs towards each other. Hands lifted overhead.

Take weight onto one leg and bend standing leg. Keep sit bones pointing down.

...under the willow tree.

13. Tree side with earth mudra

She saluted...

14. Crescent moon lunge

...the sky...

15. Low lunge twist up

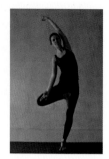

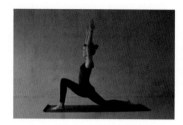

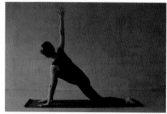

Can either rest lifted foot on floor near ankle, on shin or on thigh (not on knee). For earth mudra: thumb to ring (4th) finger in both hands.

From tree, step lifted leg back into a lunge and place knee on floor. Ensure that the front knee does not collapse inwards towards the body's midline.

Keep chest open as you twist towards front knee.

...and the earth...

16. Half plank

...perfecting...

17. Sphinx

...her movements.

18. Downward dog open hip

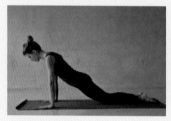

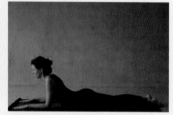

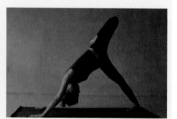

Core tight.

Hips on floor, arms at right angle, core tight, open chest.

From downward dog, lift one leg up, open at the hip, bending the knee. Both sides

19. Repeat 10–18, other side

20. Standing forward fold

21. Reach to sky

Repeat sequence 10–18, other side.

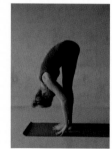

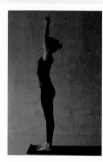

For following sequence 22–38, turn around on your mat, facing one side and then the other. From 22–29, you will be on right leg (near front of your mat). From 31–38, you will be on left leg (near back of your mat) end, facing the back of your mat. During the repeat sequence (see 39), you will turn to the other side of your mat, leading again with the right leg (near back of mat) and then left leg (near front of mat), end facing the front of your mat.

22. Standing side stretches

The goddess continued to dance...

23. Goddess pose

...as the first stars appeared in the twilight.

24. Five-pointed star

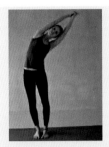

Keep both feet anchored with equal weight as you bend.

Both sides

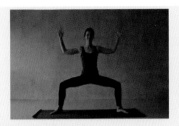

Ensure that tailbone points straight down. Open chest.

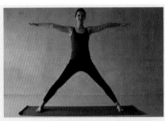

Extend through arms, legs and crown of the head.

25. Triangle

26. (Half moon – when repeating the sequence – see below)

27. Pyramid

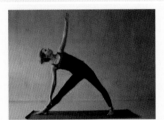

Push both hips back as you fold and open the chest with side ribs facing sky. Don't go down too far if you find chest facing floor. Can have top arm on hip rather than extended.

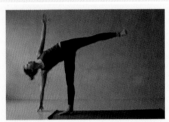

Take weight onto front leg, placing hand onto floor. Push through both feet while opening chest to the side.

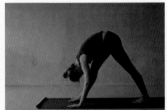

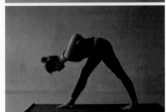

Turn towards front of mat. Ensure that hips are level. Can leave front knee slightly bent. For arms in reverse prayer, palms together behind back or just crossed behind, holding elbows.

28. Lunge runner's

Yet as she danced, her poise faltered.

29. Half squat one side

Her grace felt disgraced as her dance lost its perfection.

30. Garland squat

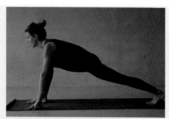

Push through back heel.

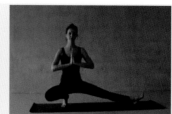

Bent knee points in same direction as foot. Can leave hands on floor if cannot balance.

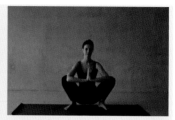

Heels down if possible, push thighs with elbows, hands in prayer. Draw pelvic floor in and keep spine long.

31. Half squat other side

32. Lunge runner's

33. Pyramid

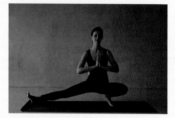

On the other side.

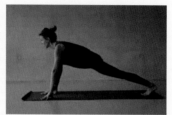

Lunge to side of bent leg. Will be turning to back of mat first time round and then second time round towards the front.

Will be facing to back of mat first time round and then second time round (during repeat sequence) towards the front.

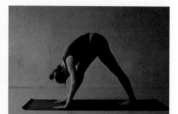

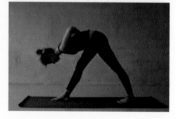

Second time with reverse prayer

34. Triangle

Cracks appeared on her golden mask...

35. (Half moon – when repeating the sequence – see below)

...as her moon dance became wilder.

36. Five-pointed star

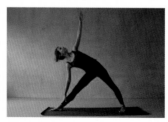

Will be facing to back of mat first time round and then second time round during the repeat sequence

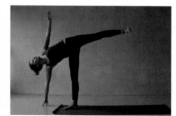

Will be facing to back of mat first time round and then second time round during the repeat sequence towards the front.

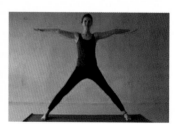

Extend through arms, legs and crown of the head.

Incandescent in the sky, the moon and stars…

37. Goddess pose

38. Standing side stretches

…reflected her flow.

39. Repeat 22–38

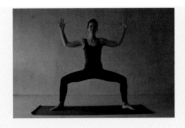

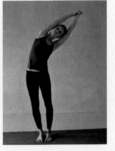

Repeat sequence 22–38 (end up facing front of mat)

Ensure that tailbone points straight down. Open chest.

End facing back of mat first time round and then second time round during the repeat sequence towards the front. Both sides.

She could feel a flame inside…

40. Fierce pose

41. Revolved fierce pose

…and was terrified.

42. Standing forward fold

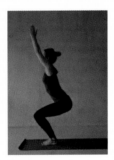

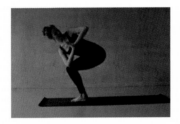

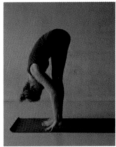

Feet and knees together, sit back, keeping spine long.

Ensure both knees are same level. Twist to one side. Can extend arms Fold from hips.
Both sides

Fold from hips. Can have knees bent.

43. Plank

A flame wavers and flickers. It had no place in the flawless grace of the goddess that she was.

44. Flowing cobra

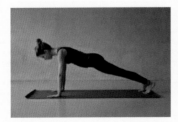

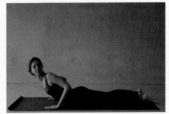

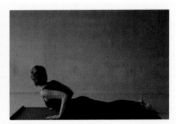

Core tight. Can have knees on the floor.

Flow one side then the other, keeping hips and feet down.

3–6 times

Her heart ached…
45. Heart pose

…torn apart because she no longer knew who she was.
46. Child pose

Seated in her temple, tear-stained and staring out into the night…
47. Bharadvaja's twist

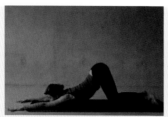

Move chest towards the floor. Can keep forehead on floor and bend arms if shoulders uncomfortable.

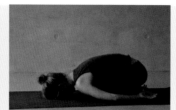

If your head does not reach the floor, you can place it on your stacked hands or fists.

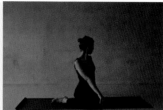

Sitting with both feet pointing to one side, ensure that hips are level. Sit one buttock on cushion if necessary to level hips. Keep spine tall as you twist away from your feet.

…she prayed.
48. Revolved gate

49. Repeat 47–48, other side

Tuning in to that desire, she turned her gaze inward…
50. Staff

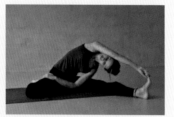

Keep both sit bones grounded and side ribs facing the sky. If bent knee uncomfortable with foot pointing backwards, do revolved head to knee pose instead.

Repeat sequence 47–48, other side.

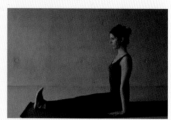

Keep both sit bones grounded and spine tall.

...towards that flickering flame.

51. Seated forward bend

Gently she let go of who she thought she needed to be.

52. Reclined butterfly pose (restorative)

As the mask finally broke, she came face to face with the flame. Warmth spread in belly and heart.

53. Supported relaxation with jnana mudra at heart and belly (restorative)

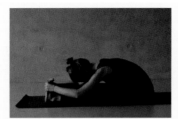

Keep both sit bones grounded. Fold from the hips. Can bend the knees if lower back is uncomfortable.

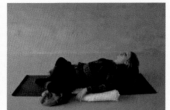

With one bolster elevated by blocks, sit on cushion and lie back on bolster, soles of the feet together. Have rolled blankets supporting arms and legs. This is meant to be a comfortable position. Lengthen exhalations, letting everything go.

Stay 3–10 min.

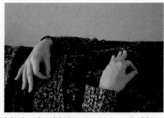

Lie back with knees supported by bolster and head on cushion. Hands in jnana mudra: thumb and index finger together. One hand on heart and other on belly. Focus on breath at these two places.

Stay 3–10 min.

She knew who she was. She was a goddess; imperfect yet perfect. She felt an immense joy, as if she had finally found her way home.

54. Chakra meditation (supported relaxation)

In above position but with arms at sides, palms facing upwards.
Meditation: visualise
At base of spine: red
At navel: orange
At solar plexus: yellow
At heart: green
At throat: light blue
At forehead: indigo
At crown of head: purple.
At each place feel bodily sensations and emotions.

Liberation

A lively young man winds himself with chains, thinking to impress others with his skill. While finishing bedecking himself, he hits his head and falls unconscious. Upon waking, he does not notice the chains that prop him up. As he starts to go about his daily work, his same daily routine, he feels himself strong and unstoppable. The chains he does not yet see provide him with added support like a suit of armour; and help him undertake his work with a strength he did not have before. Those chains are like buoys keeping him upright in the churning sea. They are like a safety harness keeping him from falling while climbing a mountain. And thus he continues through life propped up, secure but never veering off his beaten path, never noticing that he was in fact restrained.

Eventually the young man decides he wants more than his usual dreary routine and adds some variety. With the change in routine he feels at first elated but then uncomfortable. He feels pain. This feeling of pain gives him the impression he has done something wrong. And so he tries again to go back to his routine. However, everything feels wrong.

Finally he notices the chains upon him. Those chains that had once kept him strong now feel restrictive. He feels suffocated and trapped. And so he twists and tugs and pulls the chains, trying to liberate himself – to no avail. Frustrated and afraid, he laments his plight, ignorant of its cause. The more he fights, the more he finds himself caught and in pain.

Desperate, he wishes to end his life because he sees no way out of these confining chains that feel inseparable from himself. In his darkest moment of despair, he pauses and looks within. Slowly he remembers himself. It's as if light dispels the night. Those chains were of his making but were not him. And so, with slow deliberate movements, he lets go of each twist and turn of the chains until he finds himself free. With a first taste of freedom he feels as if he is flying. He has no safety net or buoy to keep him from falling, yet he can feel his own wings and the current underneath that support him.

He decides to trust those wings and that current, to trust himself; and so he starts to slowly let go of all that weighs upon him – all the routine, attitudes, behaviours and beliefs that impede his flow in life. This process is not easy and takes time; yet with each release he finds new space, he finds freedom and joy. He finds himself.

Sequence: Liberation

A lively young man…

1. Sun-piercing breath
2. Supine head to knee
3. Hip mobilisation

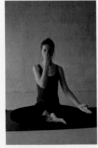

Breathe in through right nostril (closing left with ring finger) and out through left nostril (closing right with thumb). Repeat.

3 minutes

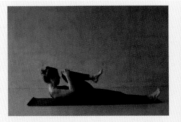

↑ Keep extended leg pressing down and core tight as you bring forehead to knee.
→ With both knees to chest, widen knees apart and then bring them back together in a circular motion. Change direction.

Both sides

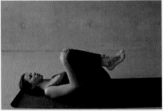

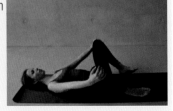

3 times each direction

...winds himself with chains...

4. Eye of the needle

5. Supine twist

6. Cat–cow

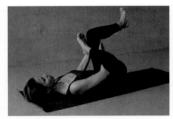

The feet should be flexed.

Both sides

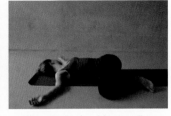

↑ Keep both shoulders on the floor.
Both sides   3–6 times

→ Inhale on A and exhale on B.

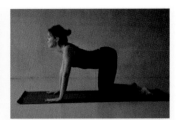

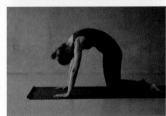

7. Dynamic cat

8. Alternate arms and legs

...thinking to impress others with his skill.

9. Downward dog (with crunches)

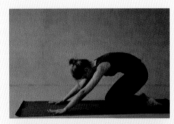

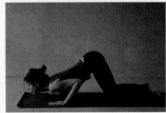

3–6 times

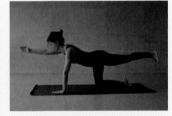

↑ Extend one leg and opposite arm, keeping your core tight.
Both sides
← Starting on all fours, A exhale, rounding back and sitting on heels, B inhale, sweeping forward chin towards floor, coming back to all fours. Repeat.

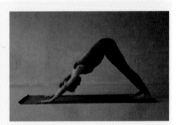

(For crunches: from downward dog, lift leg and bring knee to outside of elbow).

2 times each side

He hits his head and falls unconscious.

10. Child pose extended

Upon waking, he does not notice the chains…

11. Downward dog

12. Standing forward fold

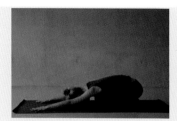

Sit on heels and extend arms forward.

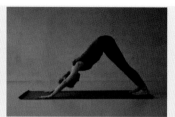

Press hips up and back. Feet hip-width apart or more. Knees can be bent to help lengthen your spine. It's fine if heels do not touch the floor.

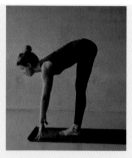

Step both feet to the front of the mat.

…that prop him up like a suit of armour.

13. Mountain pose

As he starts to go about his daily work, his same daily routine, he feels himself strong and unstoppable.

14. Sun salutation A

He decides he wants more than his usual dreary routine and adds some variety.

15. Sun salutation B

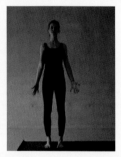

Standing tall, press down into four corners of feet. Squeeze thighs towards each other. Hands by your sides extending through fingers.

Sun A

See sun salutations.

3 times

Sun B

See sun salutations.

With the change in routine he feels at first elated…

16. Mountain pose

… but then uncomfortable.

17. Warrior I

He feels pain. This feeling of pain gives him the impression he has done something wrong.

18. Humble warrior

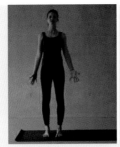

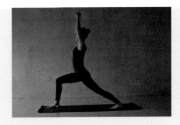

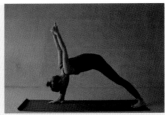

Standing tall, press down into four corners of feet. Squeeze thighs towards each other. Hands by your sides extending through fingers.

Step back one foot. Ensure that knee does not collapse inwards towards the body's midline. Your hips and torso are facing the front of your mat.

From warrior I, fold from the hips. Clasp hands behind. Arms lift away from back.

19. Vinyasa to downward dog

20. Repeat 16–19, other side

And so he tries again to go back to his routine. However, everything feels wrong.

21. Sun salutation A

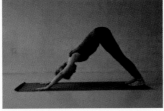

See vinyasa

Repeat sequence 16–19 other side.

Sun A

See sun salutations.

Finally he notices the chains upon him.

22. Standing twists

He feels suffocated and trapped.

23. Revolved fierce pose

And so he twists and tugs and pulls the chains, trying to liberate himself – to no avail.

24. Lunge prayer twist

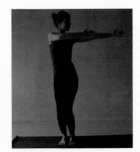

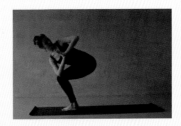

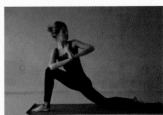

Keep both feet anchored with equal weight as you twist.
Both sides

Ensure both knees are same level. First twist to right leg (second time in repeat sequence to left leg).

From above position, step back with left leg first time (right leg second time in repeat sequence).

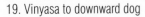

25. Vinyasa to downward dog

26. Lizard

27. Standing forward fold

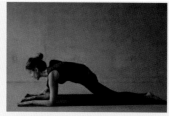

See sun salutations.

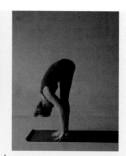

From downward dog, place right foot (left foot second time round in sequence repeat) outside of hand. No need to lower elbows to the floor if very uncomfortable. Can also lift back knee off floor.

28. Mountain pose

29. Repeat 23–28, other side

30. Forward fold with arms clasped back

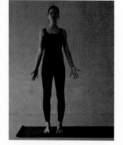

Repeat sequence 23–28, other side.

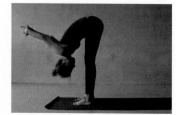

Standing tall, press down into four corners of feet. Squeeze thighs towards each other. Hands by your sides extending through fingers.

Fold from hips. Can have knees bent. Arms may not lift much from back.

31. Plank

Frustrated and afraid, he laments his plight, ignorant of its cause.

32. Side plank

The more he fights…

33. Downward dog split

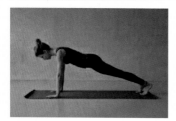

Core tight.

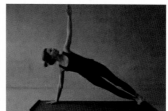

Optional – lift upper leg.

Both sides

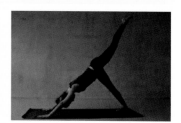

From downward dog split, place lifted foot to front of mat for next pose.

34. Warrior II

...the more he finds himself caught and in pain.

35. (Bound) side angle

36. Repeat 31–35, other side

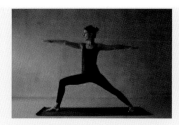 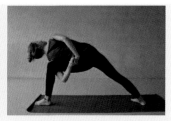

Repeat sequence 31–35, other side.

Ensure that knee does not go over ankle and is tracking second toe. Torso is open to the side.

Only bind if chest does not collapse forward.Can have elbow on knee or hand to floor (or to a block).

37. Vinyasa to downward dog

Desperate, he sees no way out of these confining chains that feel inseparable from himself.

38. Child pose

In his darkest moment of despair, he pauses and looks within.

39. Thunderbolt with uttarabodhi mudra

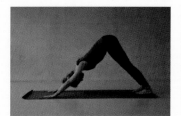 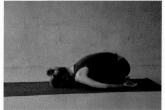 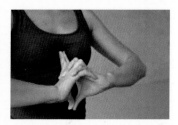

See sun salutations.

If your head does not reach the floor, you can place it on your stacked hands or fists.

Sitting on heels or other comfortable position. Hands at sternum, index fingers pointing up and thumbs down.

For following sequence 40–45: do whole sequence on one side. Then do the other as indicated in 46.

Slowly he remembers himself.

40. Downward dog (with knee to elbow)

41. Warrior II

It's as if light dispels the night.

42. Five-pointed star

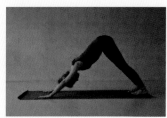 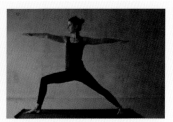 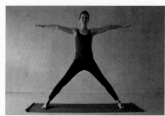

From downward dog can lift leg and bring knee to outside of elbow. Repeat. Five times one side. Keep external rotation.

Both sides

Ensure that knee does not go over ankle and is tracking second toe. Torso is open to the side.

Extend through arms, legs and crown of the head.

And so with slow deliberate movements…

43. Goddess

…he lets go of each twist and turn of the chains

44. Lizard

…until he finds himself free. He feels as if he is flying.

45. Sage Koundinya

He decides to trust himself.

46. Repeat 40–45, other side

47. Child pose

48. Hero with wrist stretch/mobilise

49. Half reclined hero

50. Staff pose

He starts to slowly let go of all that weighs upon him.

51. Seated head to knee

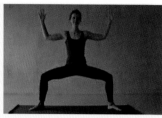

Tuck tailbone in. Draw navel to spine.

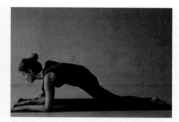

Turning to front of mat, bend into pose. Have back knee lifted.

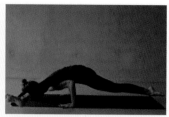

Bring front leg over upper arm and extend both. Draw navel to spine and lift back leg off floor.

Repeat sequence 40–45, other side.

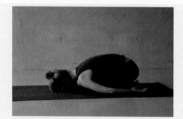

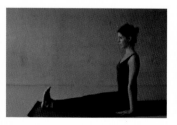

If your head does not reach the floor, you can place it on your stacked hands or fists.

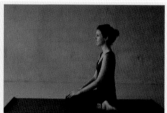

Sit between heels. Can have a cushion/block/blanket under sit bones. If not comfortable come to a comfortable seated position. Stretch and rotate wrists.

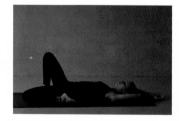

From above position lie back on to elbows or blanket (or bolster), bend one leg forward and recline back, coming only as far down as comfortable. If any pain in knee – stop!

Both sides

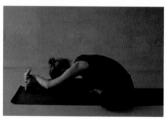

Keep both sit bones grounded and spine long.

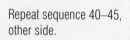

Keep both sit bones grounded. Fold from the hips over extended leg. Can bend the knee if lower back is uncomfortable.

With each release he finds new space.

52. Revolved head to knee

53. Repeat 50–52, other side

He finds freedom and joy.

54. Supine butterfly with uttarabodhi mudra

55. Supine twist

He finds himself.

56. Relaxation

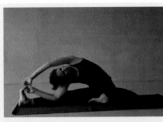

Repeat sequence 50–52, other side.

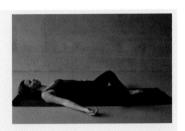

Keep both sit bones grounded and side ribs facing sky. Can bend the extended leg if necessary.

Lie with soles of the feet together and hands at chest in uttarabodhi mudra – see above.

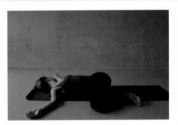 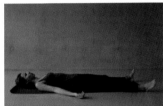

Both sides

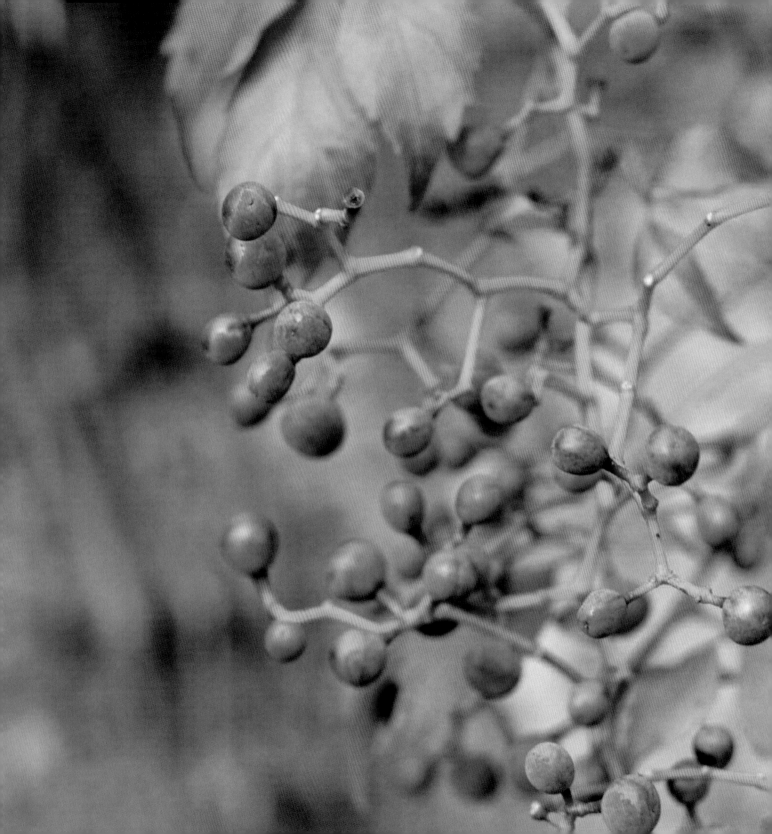

Timeless Moments Inside Out

'Life has left her footprints on my forehead. But I have become a child again this morning.
The smile, seen through leaves and flowers, is back to smooth away the wrinkles as the
rain wipes away footprints on the beach.'

Thich Nhat Hanh

'Realise deeply that the present moment is all you ever have.'

Eckhart Tolle

Her back against a smooth rock, the child delighted in the spray from the waterfall above. The soft roar of the waterfall was as loud as her beating heart when she closed her eyes to look inside. The drops from the falling water refreshed her face and body, nourishing her from the outside as the flow in her veins nourished the inside.

Eyes open, the child marvelled at the glistening drops and at the sheets like glass pouring down from the outcrop up above. A shimmering rainbow formed near the pool below: purple, indigo, blue, green, yellow, orange and red. The colours fused to her body and soul as she observed. She curved her spine, delighting in herself as rainbow.

Turning round, she gazed at the mountain brook as it wound away from the waterfall. In the distance she could see the river snaking through trees and the open plain; she could see the vast sky and the sun making its way to meet the earth. Her breath slowed, stilled by the vista ahead. Her smile spread. Looking around at the world, at nature around her, she felt aliveness well deep inside her. Each moment, each breath, was new.

As the sun set, she curled up on mossy ground next to the still pool feeling the world as a sanctuary. With the rising moon, the child gazed deep into the timeless pool. Mirrored in the surface below, her hand caressed her lined face. The reflection was that of a woman, white hair glistening in the moonlight, yet at heart a child, watching her world inside and out.

Sequence: Timeless Moments Inside Out

Equipment: 1–2 bolsters (or large pillows or piles of blankets), 3 blankets, 1 pillow, 2 blocks.
You can be inventive with the equipment. Keep the overall shape of the pose but adjust for comfort.
This is a restorative yoga sequence. Make yourself as comfortable as possible and lie in each pose for 5–15min.

Her back against a smooth rock, the soft roar of the waterfall was as loud as her beating heart when she closed her eyes to look inside.

1. Legs up the wall

She curved her spine, delighting in herself as rainbow. Purple, indigo, blue, green, yellow, orange and red. The colours fused to her body and soul as she observed.

2. Rainbow

She gazed at the mountain brook as it wound away from the waterfall. In the distance she could see the river snaking through trees and the open plain; she could see the vast sky and the sun making its way to meet the earth.

3. Mountain brook

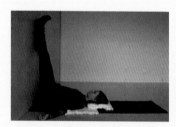

Can have back against floor or elevate hips on to a bolster by planting feet on wall, and slide bolster underneath as shown.

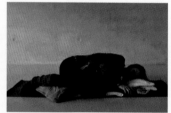

Lie with side waist over a bolster. Shoulders on a blanket and head on blanket and pillow. Can have a blanket between knees.
One side then the other.
Moving slowly to transition.

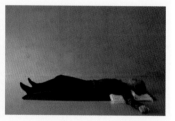

Lie with upper back on long folded blanket. Shoulders are on floor not on blanket. Head supported by blanket and knees by bolster.

Her breath slowed, stilled by the vista ahead. Looking around at the world, nature around her, she felt aliveness well deep inside her. Each moment, each breath, was anew.

4. Reclining position

As the sun set, she curled on mossy ground next to the still pool feeling the world as a sanctuary.

5. Child's pose restorative

With the rising moon, the child gazed deep into the timeless pool. The reflection was that of a woman, white hair glistening in the moonlight, yet at heart a child watching her world inside and out.

6. Moon-piercing breath

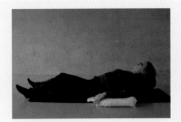

One bolster elevated by block(s), sit on cushion and recline on to bolster.
Either have knees supported by other bolster as shown or have legs crossed with knees supported by blankets. Forearms are supported by rolled blankets.

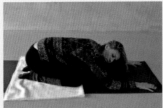

With wide knees sink back on to heels and lie over bolster. Turn head halfway through.

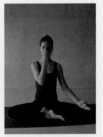

In a comfortable seated position breathe in through left nostril (closing right with thumb) and out through right nostril (closing left with ring finger). Repeat.

3–5 minutes

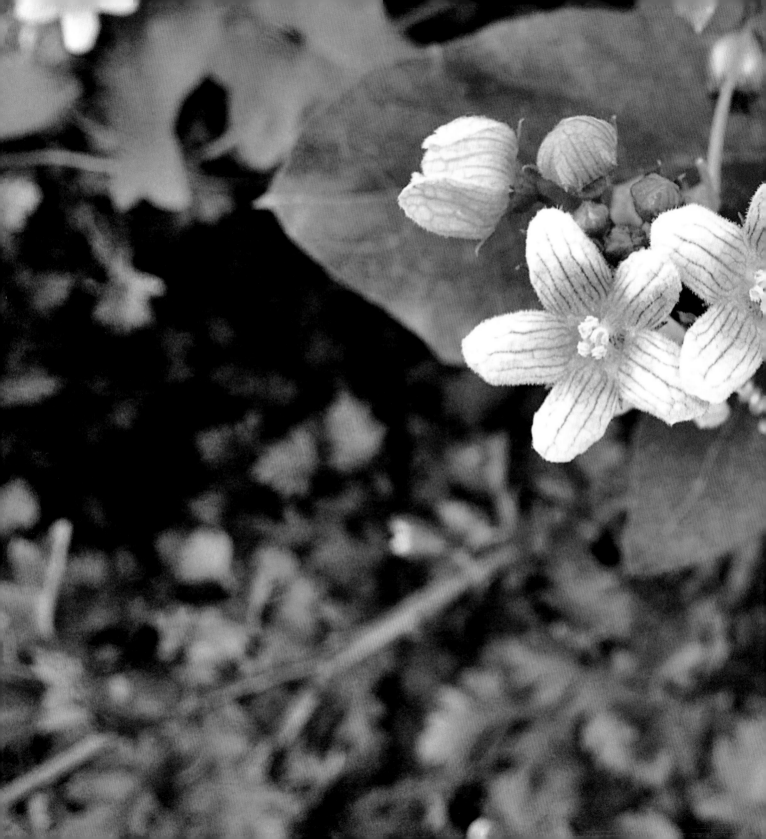

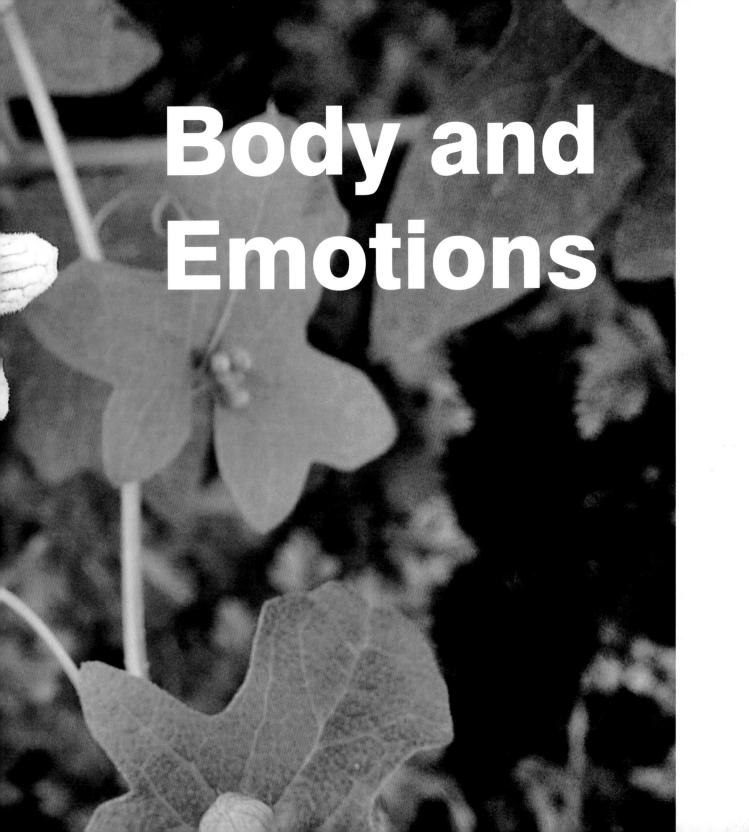

Body and
Emotions

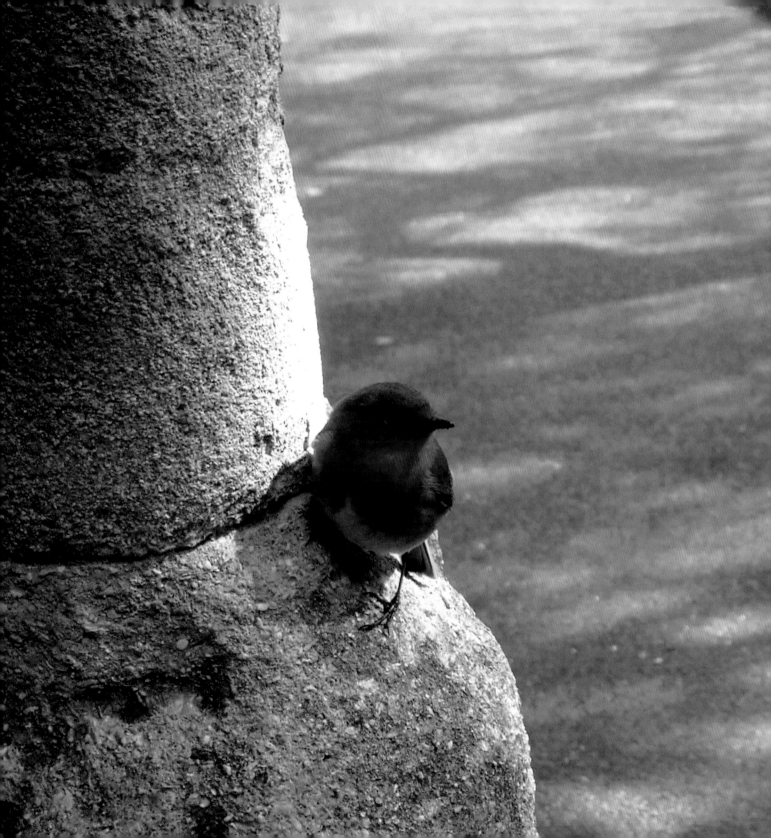

Your body's story

Sensation is the body's language

The language of the body is one of sensation, feeling and emotion. It is not a language many people can, or know how to, read very well. However, most people can understand when their bodies shout at them because they feel pain. Pain is a sign that you need to pay attention quickly and change what you are doing in order to bring relief.

But the language of the body is more rich than that: one can feel muscles 'stretch' and contract, one can feel knots in the stomach or tightness in the chest, one can feel warmth spreading through the belly and heart; and sometimes one feels nothing at all. However, you can only hear this language if you are listening, paying attention to what you feel or do not feel. Not feeling something does not necessarily mean you are doing something wrong or that there is something wrong with you. First, each body is different – for example, one person may not feel a stretch someone else would because their body is supple. Second, your brain filters sensation all the time so that you are not bombarded with every little detail that you do not need (like feeling your blood trickle through your veins).

Finally, it can take time to construct those interoceptive pathways that may have not been developed – it requires learning to have consciousness of your body and its language – or that have been shut down through trauma. Indeed, trauma can lead to one living disembodied and disconnected from one's self. This dissociation is in itself a healthy protective measure to ensure continued survival. However, over time it starts to hamper a person's ability to live life fully.

The first step to learning the language is only to pay attention to what is going on in your body with curiosity and kindness, without judging whether this is a good or bad feeling or if what you are doing is right or wrong, and without analysing what the feeling might mean. It is easier to do this through movement rather than stillness at first. Using your hands can also be useful to help you feel. For example, placing your hands on your stomach to feel the rise and fall of your breath or on a leg when extending and bending it to feel the muscles moving.

It is important to go at your own pace when investigating inner sensation because it can easily be overwhelming, especially at first. It can be like turning the radio on loudly – it can be intolerable until one gets used to it.

Understanding the meaning of the sensations will come with time. Sometimes it will come with repeated experience and you can connect the dots, so to speak. Sometimes you might want to get more information. And of course there will be times when you will just not understand and it is important to accept that too.

Sensations and feelings come and go. They pass, they change. Furthermore, you might start to notice that you have the ability to change how you feel. This is when you and your body are having a proper conversation. Starting to feel and respond to that feeling might come through doing something different with your body, whether it be changing a physical movement to change the sensation (you can twist and untwist, make a big or small movement, or stop something that is painful), doing a different physical action, e.g. going for a run to relieve stress or having a nap to feel rested, or something entirely different like talking to a friend about something that is bothering you. All this can change how you feel. You have that ability.

Sometimes it just takes some time and experimenting to figure out what you and your body need and how to go about it. And of course sometimes what you need is someone to help you get what you need (like going to get a massage or medication, for example).

Posture and feelings

How you hold yourself, your posture, affects how you feel, just as how you feel affects your posture. Standing slumped does not feel the same as standing tall, feet firmly planted on the floor. Try both these postures and see – how do you feel? Certain emotions also naturally shape the body's posture. When sad or depressed, you might be more likely to curl up or slump. When you are stressed or afraid, all your muscles tense, ready to fight or flee or freeze. When you feel exuberant, your body might feel more open with a spring in your step. It is important to respect these natural contractions and expansions, yet at the same time, if you start to get stuck in one of these, you can try working with the opposite body movement or emotion. For example, if you are stuck in sadness stand tall and open instead of slumping inwards; or if you need more relaxation, curl up. This technique is not going to help if there are serious issues that you need to deal with, of course, such as depression, grief or anxiety, but it might just help a little in getting through a day. The most important thing is that you and your body work together and not against one another.

Yoga postures also elicit feeling in the body, more than just which muscles are being stretched or engaged. Generally speaking forward folds are associated with the exhalation and are relaxing and introverting, while backbends, associated with the inhalation, are energising and extroverting. Standing poses can be grounding. You can feel strong like a warrior in warrior postures, and centred and balanced in tree posture.

However, your personal experience of these postures could in fact be quite different from these generalities. A backbend can feel liberating and joyful or, because you are exposing your chest, it can feel vulnerable and heart-wrenching or just painful. It is important to note what a posture feels like for you personally. Moreover, how you feel in a certain posture can change over time depending on how you feel overall on any given day.

Your body's story: awakening creativity

There is actually no right or wrong in how to feel in a yoga posture because your body is unique, with its own story. Indeed, life writes into and on to your body every day. It is seen through your habitual postures and feelings, your scars (internal and external) and your thought processes and constitution. Consciously embodying the story of your life rather than just thinking about it allows you to understand yourself at a deeper level. One way to start to find your story is by first noticing how you feel and how you hold yourself. Another is by finding a yoga posture or a series of postures that describe how you feel. Use your intuition and innate creativity for this; everyone will be different. For example, plank posture might describe an embodied feeling of you being overworked and stressed – or that you are feeling strong and centred!

You can also play-act with postures to give you an embodied sense of attributes rather than just thinking about them. Confidence, focus, peace are all best experienced in the body so you can find them again. Moreover, experimenting and playing are the best mediums to take the pressure away from achieving things like confidence or peace that might ordinarily seem out of reach. Einstein said that 'play is the highest form of research'. This is true because in our relaxed state of play, creativity and insight/discovery can arise more easily.

Choose a posture that has an associated meaning or attribute for you. The following are my examples; they might not have any meaning for you but they serve as illustrations. You might associate warrior I with being strong and confident – if so, see if you can become that by imagining yourself as such when you're in that posture. Eagle posture can be one of focus, like a bird watching for its prey (as long as you are stable enough in that particular form); so you can visualise yourself being focused. One of the restorative poses that fully supports your body can instil peace, like being a cat curled up on a warm rug. Give yourself permission to be silly too. You can experiment with being a triangle! Playing in this way can be tremendous fun as well as giving you an embodied sense of yourself.

Living embodied

Living embodied means being aware of how you feel in your body and being anchored there. Emotions are easier to deal with and tolerate when they can be felt in the body. Like electricity, which is more stable when earthed, emotions are more stable when they are grounded in the body. Of course some emotions are more difficult than others, but we can move with them and let them move through us when we consciously work with our selves. Physical activity is great to move things through – going for a run, for example, can help release stress. Yoga and dance also help things to flow. Whatever works for you is for you to discover. Living embodied is living in your body, not in someone else's, which means accepting your individuality.

When you live embodied you can make real decisions that are good for you. If you don't know through felt experience what feels good or bad, what nourishes your body and soul, then you can't easily make beneficial decisions. Your body is infinitely wise and it knows what you need to take care of yourself and also gives you signals – what we call instinct or intuition – to guide you. But you need to pay attention to it. You might not be able to believe that your body is wise; indeed you might believe that it easily betrays you. It is not so. Your body has adapted to its lived experience – your story – and has done everything it can for you to survive. Addictions, for example, arise as a way to survive what would otherwise be insurmountable. Sometimes those adaptations linger beyond what is necessary. However, it is always possible to change; to write a new chapter in your story. You have that power. To do that you need to join forces with yourself, to take back your power through living in the present moment, embodied. It can take time to do so because it's also about learning to love and respect yourself, your body, and that may require faith at first.

Your body tells your life story and at each moment life writes a new page on to it. You may not be able to change past chapters but you can consciously create new ones through working with life rather than letting it write your story for you.

Posture Index

Safety Guidelines

Check with a health practitioner that the exercise is appropriate and stick to any guidelines given. Below is a list of common conditions. If in doubt ask a qualified yoga practitioner. And always listen to your body.

Pregnancy and post-natal

First Trimester: only a gentle and/or restorative practice.
Second Trimester: you can continue with your regular practice in the second trimester if you have previous experience and practise modifications to all poses. No deep twists, no big backbends, no inversions, no lying on your back in relaxation poses (lie on your left side instead). Be careful not to overstretch.
Third Trimester: take specialised pregnancy yoga classes.
Post-birth: return to regular practice gently at least six weeks after giving birth (or take post-natal yoga classes). After a C-section and separated abdominal muscles, leave 12 weeks before returning to yoga practice and take extra care in twists and backbends.

Herniated disc and other back problems

Check which direction of movement is restricted or painful (and which is pain-free) and approach bending (in all directions) gradually and cautiously. Keep backbends small. No deep forward bends (especially no seated forward bends). Avoid bending forward past 90 degrees with the legs straight. In relaxation pose, keep legs bent.

Those with chronic/degenerative conditions must consult their doctor before practising yoga and (initially at least) work one-to-one with a specialised yoga therapist.

Knee problems

Be cautious in kneeling poses; modify where possible. Avoid or modify any pose that feels like the knee is under pressure (e.g. pigeon). You can make your knees more comfortable in poses where the knee is on the floor by using extra padding. Ensure correct alignment in lunge-style poses (knee does not overshoot the ankle, and should track the second toe).

Heart disease (and unregulated high blood pressure)

No inversions (or any pose where head is below heart), arm balances or (big) backbends. Modify poses so that arms are not held above the head. Do not hold poses for a long time (except restorative poses). Take it easy. Rest when necessary.

Glaucoma

No inversions or any pose where head is below heart. If medical treatment is undertaken, the patient can check with their physician if head-below-the-heart poses should be avoided indefinitely thereafter.

Carpal tunnel

Avoid/modify poses that strain or place weight on the hands or wrists (e.g. arm balances).

Arthritis

Avoid postures if joints are inflamed. No inversions for those with severe arthritic neck conditions. Modify/avoid poses that will put pressure on various joints.

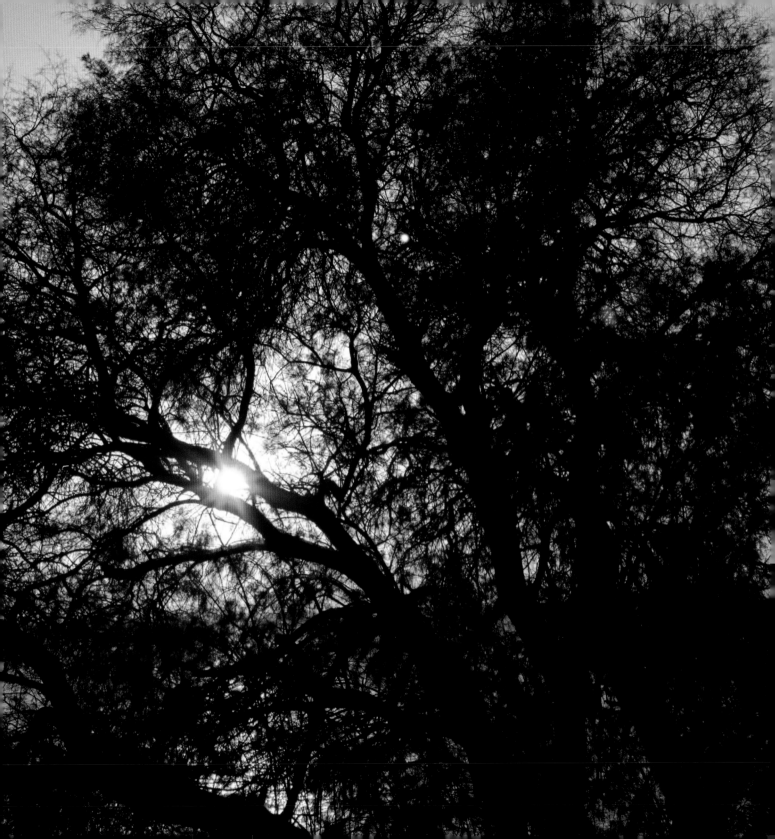

About the Author

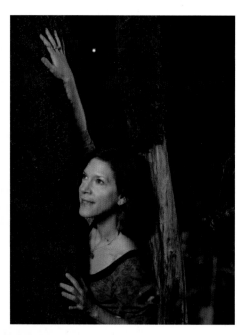

Nathalie Doswald (E-RTY®200) is a certified and experienced yoga teacher, specialising in flow, restorative and trauma-sensitive yoga. Her own personal struggles bring a rare insight and sensitivity into yoga as a practice that connects the inner spirit with the power of the mind and body.

Nathalie is both a scientist, with a PhD in Ecology and has worked with the UN on climate change and biodiversity issues; and an artist, writing stories and creating whenever possible. She is also a trained peer practitioner in mental health. Nathalie loves to mix both science and creativity in her work. She currently lives in Geneva, Switzerland, where she is founder of the association Reconnect offering yoga and meditation classes as well as workshops in her local area. She teaches yoga in English and French.

For more information see her website: www.yoga-reconnect.com

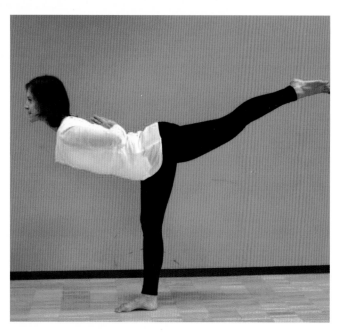

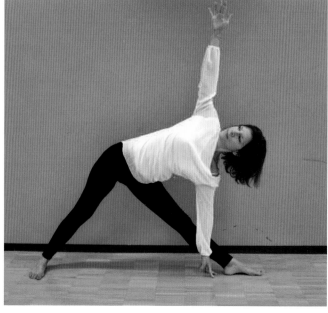

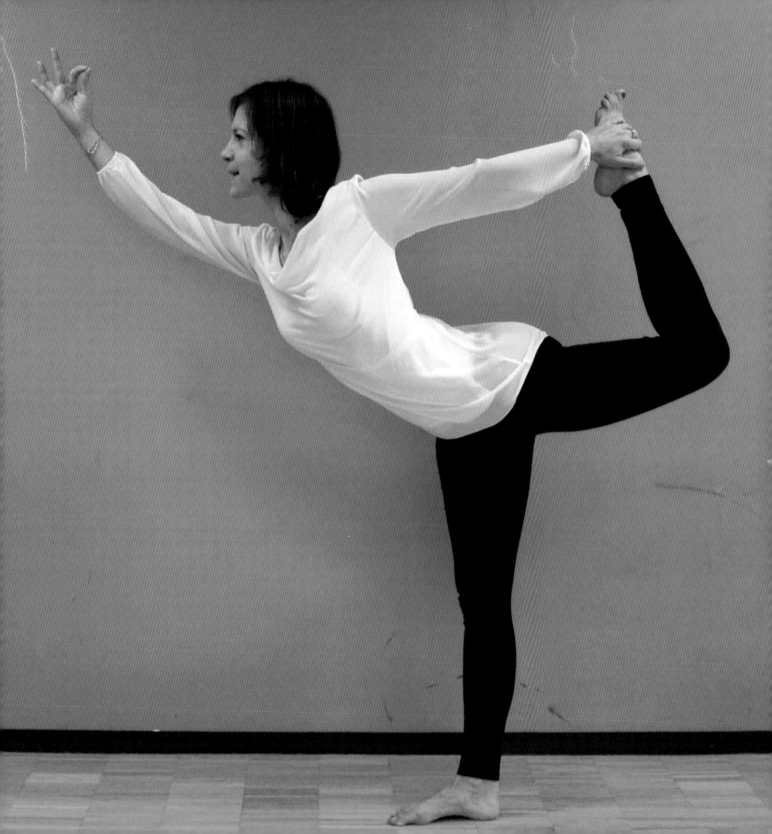